A–Z of Childhood Health Problems

Second edition

First edition published as *The A–Z Reference Book of Childhood Conditions* by Chapman & Hall 1995
Reprinted by Stanley Thornes (Publishers) Ltd 1997

Second edition published in 1999 by:
Stanley Thornes (Publishers) Ltd
Ellenborough House
Wellington Street
Cheltenham
Glos.
GL50 1YW
United Kingdom

00 01 02 03 / 10 9 8 7 6 5 4 3 2

A catalogue record for this book is available from the British Library

ISBN 0 7487 3716 2

Typeset by WestKey Limited, Falmouth, Cornwall
Printed and bound in Great Britain by Martins The Printers Ltd, Berwick upon Tweed

Contents

ACKNOWLEDGEMENTS

My thanks are due, once again, to Dr Terry Billington for the superb work done in reading this manuscript. Her comments and suggestions have been gratefully received, but any errors are entirely my own.

I would like to thank Tony Wayte at Stanley Thornes for his ever-willing availability for discussion on the format of this second edition.

As ever, my wider thanks are due to the many children and their parents who, over the years, have allowed me into their homes and lives when problems of health have arisen.

PREFACE TO THE SECOND EDITION

The original text covered conditions that mainly affect children over the age of 2 years – not that these conditions are necessarily unknown in the younger age group, but they are less likely to occur.

There are, however, health problems that can arise solely in the younger child, such as, for example, bronchiolitis, pyloric stenosis and roseola infantum. For a more complete overview of children's health problems, several of these conditions have been added. Obviously, in the space of a small volume only a selection of childhood ills can be mentioned, and these added conditions are the ones most likely to be seen in everyday situations.

In addition, sections on various generic symptoms, such as 'headache' and 'rashes' have also been added. So, again, while the list of possible causes of each of these signs and symptoms is not necessarily exhaustive, clues as to possible underlying factors can be gained. It must be stressed, however, that children can become seriously ill in a very short space of time, and delay in obtaining medical help can be dangerous.

A short discussion on the current schedule of immunization procedures has also been added. This is, of course, subject to change in the light of new knowledge and/or new vaccines becoming available.

It is hoped that this extended version will be of greater value to a wider range of readers having the daily care of children. (The new title is, hopefully, also more 'user-friendly' than its predecessor!)

Patricia Gilbert
May 1998

Preface to the First Edition

Children, as well as adults, become ill. Any time or place can herald the onset of sometimes severe or even life-threatening illness. For instance, a child may set off for school seemingly perfectly fit and well. But by midday the child can be burning with fever, in severe pain or maybe in need of urgent hospital admission.

Anyone having the care of children, and certainly those many dedicated people who spend their lives working with children, needs a basic knowledge of childhood illnesses. As well as knowledge of emergency treatment for a variety of conditions, knowledge of prevention and the spread of infectious disease, plus the natural history of the illness, is valuable in the working situation. Teachers, play-group leaders, nursery staff, social workers as well as those people more intimately concerned with the care of sick children need a quick, ready reference for unexpected events that may occur during the course of a working day. Parents, including the many devoted foster-parents having the care of a number of children throughout their lives, can also require a readily available source of reference.

It is hoped that this volume will prove of value in this context. The alphabetical arrangement facilitates rapid access to the appropriate condition. The index is also comprehensively arranged to allow for specific symptoms to lead the reader to the most likely cause of the problem.

Long-term implications as well as possible later complications are also to be found under the appropriate heading. The emphasis is on the practical day-to-day management of the many common – and some less common – illnesses affecting children.

Selection of the conditions included has been based on two criteria. Firstly, the condition under discussion is relatively common, and one from which many children will suffer during the course of their early lives. This includes the common infectious illnesses such as gastroenteritis, chickenpox and tonsillitis, for example, as well as such diverse conditions as bed-wetting, warts and eczema. Secondly, the condition is less common, but is one which it is important to understand in order that the child can be helped to lead as normal a life as is possible within the limitations of the condition. This group includes such conditions as diabetes, epilepsy and coeliac disease as well as other possibly less well-known conditions such as Perthes' disease and epidermolysis bullosa. All these conditions can be found amongst both schoolchildren and their younger brothers and sisters.

A glossary of some unavoidable medical terms has been added at the end of the book and, where appropriate, names and addresses of self-help groups have been included at the end of each specific section.

It is hoped that this book will be a valuable 'working companion' to the many people who have the vital day-to-day care of the up-and-coming generation.

SPECIAL FEATURES OF CHILDREN'S DISEASES

Children are not 'mini-adults'. They are special people in their own right with special problems and needs. This is probably never so obvious as when they become ill – for a number of reasons.

PATTERNS OF ILLNESS

This, in everyone, can be broken down into five basic causative factors.

Disease (or 'lack of ease') can be due to a **congenital** problem. This includes all the multitude of syndromes, more and more of which are being recognized, described and classified with every passing week. A congenital disease is one that is present from birth and often has its roots in a genetic or chromosomal defect. These defects may be inherited from either parent or can be the result of a mutation during cell division. Examples of this type of problems can range from the serious to the relatively minor. For example, Down's syndrome is the result of a chromosomal abnormality, the results of which have far-ranging effects for the child and his/her family throughout life. A further example of a congenital disorder is haemophilia, in which direct family links can often be followed. This disease affects only males, but is passed on through the female line. As with Down's syndrome, the effects of this congenital problem are felt throughout life.

Relatively minor congenital problems can also occur, such as, webbing of the toes, or an extra digit on one hand. (Look in old paintings for the long sleeves that hide the sixth digit on Anne Boleyn's hand!) These latter findings are unlikely to cause any significant problems in later life, but make a fascinating part of the study of family history.

Many congenital problems are obvious either at birth or certainly during the first few weeks of life. With accurate diagnosis and sensitive long-term advice and discussion, parents can be helped to come to terms with their child's congenital condition. Also, of great importance, they can be shown ways to help their child grow to reach his/her full potential with the help of other people concerned with the care of the child – nursery staff and teachers bringing their own special expertise.

Secondly, **infections** of all kinds play a large part in the illness of children. Newborn babies arrive in the world with some immunity to the infections which surround us all the time. This immunity is passed on from mother to child both prenatally and in breast-milk, provided, of course, that the mother herself has contracted and overcome the specific disease. For example, if a mother has never suffered an attack of measles (but remember that attacks of infection can be subclinical) she will have no antibodies available in her body to pass on to her baby. So the baby will be susceptible to this infection should it be met. As the baby grows and matures, immunity to infectious disease will be gained. But to do this s/he will, of necessity, have to suffer from the infection. This gaining of natural immunity makes up a large part of the illnesses of childhood.

Before the advent of active immunization against a number of infections, many children were laid low – sometimes with fatal results – by these so-called 'childhood infections'. Today's children in the western world are fortunate indeed to have the vaccines available to prevent large-scale epidemics (which occurred with monotonous regularity) of such diseases as diphtheria and polio and, until fairly recently, measles, mumps and rubella.

But infections such as sore throats, headaches and runny noses still abound, and lucky is the child – and his/her parents – who escapes with only a few of these episodes in the preschool and early school years. Unfortunately, unlike the childhood infections such as mumps and chickenpox, the bacteria/viruses causing the common cold undergo subtle changes every year or so. So, the immunity gained one year against one specific type of infection is not effective against the infections occurring the following year. Thus the seemingly endless round of upper respiratory infections persists throughout the early years of childhood.

Other more serious forms of infection, such as meningitis, are also hazards to be remembered when a child becomes ill. Immunization has recently become available against one particular form of meningitis. But there are a number of other infective agents that can cause this serious disease.

Again, today's children are fortunate that powerful antibiotics are available to be used in the fight against infectious disease. But these drugs are effective only against bacterial infections (with very few exceptions). Infections with viruses are not helped by antibiotics.

So, infections of all kinds probably account for much of the illness during the childhood years. And, in spite of modern medicines and treatments, long-term complications – and fatalities – do still occur.

Then, new growths or **tumours** cause illness in children as well as in adult life. Cancers of all kinds affect children, leukaemia (a cancer of the blood) perhaps being the commonest and best known of these. The types of tumour encountered in childhood differ from the adult pattern. Some are similar, but there are a number of cancers that are specific to childhood, such as Wilms' tumour and retinoblastoma.

This group of illnesses must always be remembered when a child is ill for an unusually long time. They are now second only to accidents as a cause of death in the 1–15 age group. In these circumstances, quick diagnosis and treatment must be undertaken for the best chance of cure.

The fourth main category of disease is the **degenerative** diseases. These are far more commonly seen in the older generation, but occasionally children are affected by this type of condition. Examples are the degenerative brain disorders such as the mucopolysaccharide diseases – Hunter's and Hurler's syndromes – and other conditions with a biochemical basis.

Many of these diseases have a genetic basis, and they must always be remembered if a child, of school age or during the toddler years, shows a fall-off of skills that have already been learned.

Finally, **allergic** disease is a common cause of illness in childhood. Examples of this type of disorder are the trio of asthma, eczema and hay-fever – so often seen in one form or another in members of the same family. In this group can also be placed certain types of food allergy, such as the allergy to the protein in wheat seen in children (and adults) with coeliac disease. Allergy to cow's milk (often a temporary phase only) as well as other food allergies are also an important aspect of childhood illness.

(**Accidents** of all kinds, from accidental poisoning to road traffic accidents, are a further important cause of distress and 'dis-ease' in children. Their cause, prevention and treatment are a subject on their own.)

TYPES OF DISEASE

Types of disease, as already hinted at, can be quite different from those seen in adults and specific to the childhood years. The osteochondrites in which certain bones (Perthes' disease affecting the hips, for example) become weakened and friable, causing pain and loss of use, are good examples of this. No such condition is seen in adult life. The specific tumours – Wilms' tumour and retinoblastoma – are further examples of conditions found only in childhood.

Further pitfalls in diagnosis are also caused by the ways in which children react to disease. For instance, an adult with tonsillitis will be only too well aware that his throat is sore and is the basic reason why he is feeling unwell. A child with a similar condition can easily throw her mother off the scent by complaining of abdominal pain, and make no mention at all of her throat even though this can be a fiery red and very obviously infected. Maybe this is because the child has not developed, as yet, the verbal skills to accurately pinpoint pain, or maybe it is because different physiological patterns occur in childhood. Whatever the reason, knowledge of these factors will enable the true diagnosis (and hence appropriate treatment) to be made more rapidly.

Children also react to disease, such as an infection, more rapidly than do adults. All child-carers are aware that children can wake perfectly fit and bubbling over with life and energy. But by lunch-time, they can be feverish, in pain and, on occasions, severely ill. Fortunately, the reverse also holds true. Children can bounce back to health in a surprisingly short time.

STAGE OF DEVELOPMENT

The stage of development reached when a child suffers a specific disease is also of importance when the long-term effects are being considered. For example, a severe infection of one kind or another contracted during the early stages of speech development can cause marked delay in the acquisition of this skill. If a similar infection is acquired at a much later date – 10 years of age or so, when speech and language are fully developed – there will be little or no effect on this skill.

Similarly a child's other developmental 'milestones' – such as the motor one of walking and the finer motor skills, such as hand dexterity – can be affected more seriously by an illness during the critical months of development of the particular skill.

All in all, disease in children can be a minefield of diagnostic pitfalls! But how satisfying and rewarding can be the results of correct detection of the clues – leading to appropriate treatment and cure of many of the childhood ills. Heartache, too, can regretfully occur when a disease is found to be, in the present state of knowledge, incurable. But at least the child's life can be made as comfortable and fulfilling as possible by accurate knowledge of the natural history and course of the condition.

ACNE

INCIDENCE

The exact incidence of acne is not documented, but the condition is so common in adolescence as to be almost a normal part of growing-up. Fortunate indeed are the adolescents who escape with no signs of acne at all. Boys are more commonly affected than girls.

While adolescence is by far the most usual time of life for acne to occur, newborn babies are occasionally seen with the typical lesions, usually on the cheeks. No treatment is necessary at this early age, as the acne will disappear spontaneously by around 6 weeks.

Again, acne can make its first appearance at around 3 months of age, also most often only on the cheeks. At this age it can be more of a persistent problem, and will need treatment if it is to clear within the next 2 years. Often there is a strong family history of acne, and these children frequently have a return of the typical rash later in life, most commonly in the adolescent years.

HISTORY

Acne has been described in the literature from time immemorial. The word 'acne' comes from the Greek word *acme*, meaning the pinnacle, or prime, of life. An apt description of adolescence – physically at least!

CAUSATION

The rash of acne arises from the sebaceous glands. The commonest areas of the body to be affected are the face, back and chest. The sebaceous glands secrete a substance known as sebum. This substance largely consists of fatty chemicals that perform the vital function of lubricating the skin. With the appearance of acne, a number of changes take place in these glands:

- there is an increase in the amount of sebum produced;
- there is an increase in the fatty acid content of the sebum;
- the lining of the ducts become thickened to produce the typical comedones (or 'blackheads') of acne (the blackening is due to an increase in pigment, and not to dirt!);
- a specific bacteria causes inflammation to occur around the glands.

These changes, occurring in varying degrees in different people, give rise to the typical rash of acne.

There are a number of underlying factors which, in turn, cause these changes to take place.

- At puberty there is an increase in the male **hormones**, especially in boys. Girls also have a proportion of male hormone in their bodies, and at puberty there can be a temporary imbalance in the proportions of male and female hormones.
- In girls, **fluid retention** can be a problem premenstrually. This is thought to have a bearing on the worsening of acne during the premenstrual days.

These two factors are the most important causes of acne, the temporary hormonal imbalance being the most important.

Other factors include the following.

- Certain items of **diet** have been said to affect the severity of the lesions in some boys and girls. Chocolate, coffee and nuts have all been implicated, but this is an individual variation.
- Some specific **oils** used in certain industries – and even the oil used in some cosmetics – can lead to a worsening of the rash. DDT and some weedkillers have also been implicated in the onset of acne.
- **Drugs** such as the steroids, some anticonvulsant drugs and some of the combined types of oral contraceptives can also be triggering causes.
- The **time of year** also appears to have a bearing on the severity of the rash; summer light having a good effect. Acne is often at its worst during the winter months.

CHARACTERISTICS

There are two main types of acne described – in addition to the type seen in young children.

Acne vulgaris is by far the most common type. Around 40% of boys have some degree of this type of acne between 17 and 19 years of age. Girls seem to suffer from acne at a slightly earlier age – around 16 to18 – probably coinciding with the optimum time of hormonal imbalance.

The skin of sufferers often tends to be more greasy than normal, because of the increased production of sebum. In severe cases the rash can leave scars that remain visible throughout life – the scars seen on the back of the neck in some adult men being a permanent reminder of their youth.

Acne conglobata is a severe form of acne in which the spots are so numerous that they become confluent, with many inflamed and cystic nodules filled with pus. In extreme cases there can be associated fever and general feelings of ill-health. This is especially common in the tropics.

MANAGEMENT

This can require long-term sensitive handling during the adolescent years when it is important – in both boys and girls – to look as good as possible. They should be reassured that their spots will eventually clear, but meanwhile there are a number of treatments that can be tried.

- It is important to keep the skin as **clean** as possible to reduce the incidence of infection of the spots with the bacteria specific to acne. Holding a hot damp flannel to the face – or bending over a bowl of steaming water – will open up the pores. If this is followed by gentle washing with unperfumed soap, infection will be reduced to a minimum. This should be done two or three times a day.
- There are a number of **proprietary preparations** for application to the rash on the market for the control of acne. Most of these act by dissolving the plug of dried skin cells in the spots (or comedones) as well as reducing the greasiness of the skin. **Vitamin A**, manufactured as a cream, can also be helpful.
- **Sunlight** has a beneficial effect on acne. Ultraviolet light has been tried as a treatment, but is found to be less effective than natural sunlight. But it is useful in the winter months when natural sunlight is at a minimum.
- **Oxytetracycline** or **erythromycin** in tablet form is also helpful in some severe cases of acne. It is often necessary to take this form of medication on a long-term basis as it can be several months before any improvement is seen. (Tetracycline interferes with the action of some forms of contraceptive pill and must not be given in pregnancy. So care must be taken with this form of treatment in adolescent girls.)
- Other medicaments are available to treat extremely severe cases of acne. These must be given with care, and must be very carefully monitored as serious side-effects can occur.

A number of ways of controlling the condition may have to be tried before finding a treatment that suits the individual person with acne. Reassurance that the rash will eventually disappear is an all-important ingredient in the treatment. It must be stressed that any treatment given must be continued on a long-term basis.

PREVENTION

There is no known prevention for acne, apart from choosing to be born into a family that has no history of acne! Scrupulous cleanliness of the affected areas, and persistence with treatment, are the best ways of controlling the condition.

THE FUTURE

Acne in adulthood is rare, although it is thought that around 1% of men and 5% of women have some degree of acne in middle life.

SELF-HELP GROUP

The Acne Support Group
PO Box 230
Hayes
Middlesex, UB4 0UT
Tel. 0181 561 6868.

Anorexia nervosa

Alternative name

Eating disorder.

Incidence

Anorexia nervosa is most commonly found in adolescent girls, but the condition is by no means unknown in younger children. Also, in a recent survey, it was found that one quarter of the cases in this younger age group were boys.

In the younger age group (8–14 years of age) the condition can reach a dangerous state without recognition – probably because anorexia nervosa is considered to be solely a disease of older girls.

The incidence of this condition appears to be on the increase in western countries.

Causation

In adolescent girls psychological factors are probably the prime instigators in the onset of anorexia nervosa. Today's fashions all shout the message that 'thin is beautiful', and the fashion-conscious teenager will respond to this. Anorexia sufferers also have a distorted image of their own body shape – insisting that they are fat, ugly and 'overweight' when, in fact, their bones stand out starkly and unattractively.

At a deeper level, fear of adulthood with all its responsibilities and stresses can subconsciously lead the adolescent into ways of keeping a childish anatomy and physiology. The menarche – around 12–14 years – is a definitive sign of approaching maturity, and this is the age when anorexia commonly begins.

Over-close family relationships are also considered to have a possible bearing on the aetiology of anorexia nervosa. This especially applies to a close, intrusive mother–daughter relationship.

Children with this condition also tend to be perfectionists who worry about many aspects of everyday living.

Characteristics

The onset of anorexia nervosa is usually insidious, the youngster using all kinds of tactics so that parents will be unaware of how little s/he is eating. Food is hidden, small helpings frequently requested, meals are avoided, strange diets are tried and, later in the disease, the sufferer will induce vomiting and/or use excessive doses of laxatives.

The physical features of this disease are very non-specific. It is when these features are combined with other behavioural abnormalities that anorexia nervosa should be suspected.

Physical characteristics

- **Weight loss.** This, of course, is the most important sign. In children during the actively growing years, it must be remembered that lack of normal weight gain is also a significant factor. The ratios of the weight and height for age must be taken into consideration.
- **Obvious lack of appetite.** Most children from 8 years upwards have healthy appetites, unless they are suffering from an intercurrent infection or some other disorder. A transient anorexia often follows such events, but usually soon picks up again. After a long day at school or pursuing some holiday activity, the evening meal is generally consumed with relish. Children with anorexia will make all kinds of excuses for avoiding this meal.
- The child may complain of **abdominal pain or discomfort**, and may make this an excuse for not eating.
- Complaints of **tiredness and dizziness** may also be features of this condition.

On examining the child, features other than thinness and a poor weight (in relation to age and height) are seen:

- **cold hands and feet** due to poor circulation;
- a **dry skin**;
- **low blood pressure**;
- a **slow pulse**, and, later on in the disease, **slow, deep breathing**.

(In the late stages of the disease the child's breath will have the characteristic smell of acetone (pear-drops). This is due to the breakdown of body tissue as a result of the virtual starvation.)

Behavioural characteristics

- **Moodiness** with depressive thoughts and outlook.
- **Loss of interest** in most aspects of living, including activities previously much enjoyed.
- There is often a marked interest in some aspects of **food**, including such emotive issues as animal rights and hunger in the world.
- There may be a **clinical depression** in association with these other manifestations of anorexia nervosa.

Bulimia nervosa is an allied condition, and can coexist with anorexia nervosa. Here the sufferer will 'binge', or overeat, and then induce vomiting. Excessive purgatives can also be taken in an effort to counteract the overeating.

Ultimately, when fluids are being refused as well as food, **dehydration** can occur. Signs of this serious condition are sunken eyes, a weak pulse, a low blood pressure and a decreased output of urine. The child is then seriously ill and in urgent need of treatment. Death can occur – and does in some 5% of children with severe anorexia nervosa. Death can be due to hypothermia, an infection that the weakened body is unable to counteract or irreversible changes in the body chemistry.

Management

Treatment for severe anorexia nervosa is difficult and long-term. Often a period of hospital admission – preferably in a specialized unit – is needed. The initial aim is to **rehydrate** and **re-feed** the child until a normal pattern of eating has been re-established. This obviously cannot happen overnight – the child who has eaten practically nothing will need to increase intake at a slow, but steady, rate. The help of a dietician is valuable in ensuring a balanced diet.

In very severe cases, where the child is adamant that s/he will not eat, nasogastric feeding may need to be undertaken as a last resort during the initial stages of treatment. (Occasionally, the suggestion that this might be done is sufficient to start the child eating again.)

Once this initial physical hurdle has been overcome, it is necessary for the basic cause of the original onset of the anorexia to be tackled. A child psychiatrist with a special interest in anorexic children is of prime importance in the liaison that must take place between paediatrician, general practitioner, health visitor, dietician and others concerned with helping the child and the family.

Treatment for any underlying depressive disease with antidepressant drugs must also be undertaken.

The future

A **return of the anorexia nervosa** at times of stress – examinations, boy/girl relationships, etc. – can occur, and must be contained by early specialized help. Depending at what stage of growth the anorexia has occurred, **final adult height** may be adversely affected. This is particularly likely if the condition has occurred during the time of a growth spurt.

Later, **fertility** may be affected in girls. This is due to possible changes to the ovaries and uterus during the time of poor nutrition. The incidence of this effect is not fully known. **Osteoporosis** is also thought to be a possible late effect of earlier anorexia nervosa. The early teenage years are a time when a healthy bony skeleton is laid down. If virtual starvation at this time precludes this, adequate later bone density may be poor. Again, this effect is not fully understood.

Anorexia nervosa can be a difficult condition firstly to diagnose and secondly to treat. Best results are obtained with early help before body changes become too pronounced or severe.

SELF-HELP GROUP

Eating Disorders Association
1st floor, Westsum House
103 Prince of Wales Road
Norwich
Norfolk, NR1 1DW
Tel. 01603 621414.

APPENDICITIS

INCIDENCE

Appendicitis is no more common in childhood than in adult life. A recent national survey in the UK found that around three or four children in every 1000 suffered from appendicitis every year. The condition is seen at any age, but is more usually found over the age of 5 years. Appendicitis is an emergency at any age, but especially so in children. The appendix is a small, finger-like projection from the caecum – a part of the large intestine situated in the right lower part of the abdomen. In childhood the wall of this vestigial organ is thin, and so rupture can occur more readily. Rupture leads to **peritonitis**. This is a serious condition where the abdominal cavity becomes inflamed and infected as a result of the contents of the bowel spilling out in this body cavity. Unless the appendix is removed surgically the condition can be fatal. In fact, there were four deaths from appendicitis in Scotland as recently as the late 1970s.

HISTORY

Probably the best known historical fact related to appendicitis is King Edward VII's appendicectomy. This operation, away back in the early days of the 20th century, was one of the first to be successfully performed in the UK.

CAUSATION

In plant-eating animals the appendix fulfils a digestive function. In the human this organ is merely a vestigial remnant, fulfilling no useful purpose at all. Inflammation occurs in this part of the intestine with specific bacteria that are normally present. It is when either a kink develops in the appendix itself or when something obstructs the lumen, that problems can arise.

The offending obstruction can be anything from, for example, an apple-pip to a toothbrush bristle! More frequently, however, hardened food material is found to be the probable cause of the obstruction.

Initially the inflammation is localized in the appendix, but surrounding lymph-glands and other abdominal tissues quickly become involved. It is this reaction that gives rise to the typical pain of appendicitis.

CHARACTERISTICS

The correct diagnosis of acute abdominal pain in children is notoriously difficult. Appendicitis can be just one of the many causes of this common childhood symptom. Much experience is necessary to unravel all the clues. But it is vital that an acute inflammation of the appendix is not missed. In fact, it is preferable that a normal appendix is removed than an inflamed – and potentially dangerous – one is missed.

Typically, the signs of appendicitis are as follows.

- There is a sudden onset (over an hour or so) of **colicky abdominal pain**. This pain can be continuous or, alternatively, come in spasms. The pain usually starts around the area of the umbilicus. In adults, the pain typically moves, after a short time, to the right lower part of the abdomen. This can also occur in children, but frequently the child describes the main pain as remaining in the centre of the abdomen. If the appendix is in an unusual position behind the main bowel, the pain is felt more in the loin region.
- Most children with appendicitis have at least one episode of **vomiting**.
- **Diarrhoea** is also a relatively common feature at first in childhood appendicitis. This is then followed by constipation.
- There is commonly, but not invariably, a **rise in temperature**.
- The child will prefer to **lie still** and curled round in an attempt to reduce the pain.

INVESTIGATIONS

There are no specific investigations that need to be made to confirm the diagnosis of appendicitis, although **ultrasound scans** may be used as an aid to diagnosis. It is, however, wise to **test the child's urine** to exclude a urinary infection as the cause of the pain.

MANAGEMENT

The treatment for appendicitis is an operation to remove the appendix. Even if, at operation, the appendix is found not to be inflamed, it is removed to prevent trouble at any later date. A short stay in hospital is necessary following surgery. If the child has been seriously ill prior to operation, intravenous fluids may be necessary for a short while during and after the operation. Dissolvable stitches are used, so that there need be no fear for the child of their removal – as was the case a decade or so ago.

Early **movement** is encouraged, and the child is allowed to play. Children are very good at judging the limits of their abilities under such circumstances.

A normal **diet** can be given as soon as the child asks for food.

Schooling can usually be resumed after 2 or 3 weeks following an appendicectomy. This will depend, of course, on how ill the child has been prior to surgery. No restrictions need to be put on activities, but any complaints of pain after physical activities should always be fully investigated, and quieter pursuits advised for a short time.

COMPLICATIONS

There are few complications to a straightforward appendicectomy, but occasionally **infection** can occur locally around the incision. This is readily cured with antibiotics.

THE FUTURE

There are no long-term problems following appendicitis. Indeed, if the appendix has been removed, appendicitis need never again be considered as a possible cause of future abdominal pain!

Arthritis

Alternative names

Juvenile chronic arthritis (the name most commonly used); juvenile rheumatoid arthritis; Still's disease. (The two latter names are rarely used. This follows review of the classification of this disease, necessary because of the wide variation in its manifestations.)

Incidence

There are no exact figures available for the incidence of juvenile chronic arthritis, but it is probably the most common of the connective disorders seen in childhood. It is seen in all countries of the world, and is thought probably to have an incidence similar to that of diabetes in childhood, i.e. around two children in every 1000. So while it is not a particularly common disease, affected children will need much monitoring and care.

The usual age of onset is below 5 years, but the condition can occur in any age group throughout childhood. Both sexes are equally affected. (This form of rheumatic arthritis must not be confused with acute rheumatic fever, which was a far more common, and serious, disease of childhood half a century or so ago. Acute rheumatic fever is also primarily a disease of connective tissue, and can have arthritis as part of its symptomatology. There is a strong association between acute rheumatic fever and infection with a particular type of streptococcal bacterium, which is not the case with juvenile chronic arthritis. The incidence of rheumatic fever has declined as a result of three factors:

- better living conditions, which diminish infection rates;
- the advent of the penicillins, which are active against streptococci;
- a decline in the virulence of the specific *Streptococcus* bacteria.)

History

It was Dr George Frederic Still who first described the condition (or group of conditions) now known as juvenile chronic arthritis in 1896. Until fairly recently the condition was referred to as Still's disease. It is since the specific subtypes have been classified more stringently that the disease has been renamed juvenile chronic arthritis.

Causation

Juvenile chronic arthritis is part of the wide group of diseases that affect the connective tissues of the body. Several factors are thought to be involved in the causation of the disease – firstly, there is probably some genetic predisposition to this group of diseases; secondly, an autoimmune process (in which the body starts attacking its own tissues); and, finally, added infection may play a part in the onset.

CHARACTERISTICS

Arthritis and rheumatism are wide-ranging disorders of connective tissue, there being over 200 different types known. Several of these can affect children. Three of the more common modes of onset, and subsequent progress, of the disease will be described.

Systemic juvenile chronic arthritis

This type of arthritis begins with a feverish illness. The **fever** occurs daily and can be as high as 40.5°C. This fever usually resolves at some time during the day, only to return again within the next 24 hours. This intermittent pattern can make the diagnosis difficult to differentiate from a number of other diseases that have an intermittent fever as part of the initial symptomatology.

All the attendant signs and symptoms associated with fever occur – **a rapid pulse, shivery feelings, lack of appetite** and **irritability. Glands** in the neck, armpit and groin become swollen and tender. A **rash**, of a typical coppery-red colour, also affects some children during these initial stages of the illness. This rash is especially noticeable following a hot bath, but is not an irritating one.

At this early stage, **arthritis** with tender swollen joints may be completely absent – only to appear a few weeks, or even months, later. (This fact can, of course, make for great difficulties in diagnosis.)

Investigations for systemic onset disease

While there are no specific tests for juvenile chronic arthritis, **blood tests** will show abnormalities.

- The **white blood cell** count is high.
- **Anaemia** is usually present.
- The **erythrocyte sedimentation** rate is raised. (This is a non-specific test that is positive in any condition where there is any degree of inflammation, due to any cause.)

All these findings can be due to any number of other conditions, and so are of no specific help in diagnosis, but, of course, all give added clues.

To add to the difficulties, a positive rheumatoid factor, found in the blood in other types of onset of this disease, is rarely found when the disease has this acute systemic onset.

Polyarticular juvenile chronic arthritis

This is perhaps an easier onset from the diagnostic point of view for various reasons.

- A number of **joints** will be **painful, red** and **swollen**. The joints involved in this process are usually the smaller ones of the body – wrists, finger joints, ankles and, at times, knees. The specialized joints in the neck (those with limited movement) can also be involved. Because of this the child may complain of neck pain, and may be holding his/her head over to one side. The temporomandibular joint (concerned with opening the jaw) is also often involved. For this type of juvenile chronic arthritis to be diagnosed, five or more joints should be involved in the disease process.
- A **low-grade fever** can also be present, but is quite unlike the variable, spiking fever pattern associated with the acute systemic onset of the condition.
- Swelling of the **lymph glands** may also occur, but not to such a marked extent as with the systemic-type onset.

Investigations (polyarticular type)

A **blood test** specific for the rheumatoid factor can be done, but again can be somewhat unhelpful – some children will have a positive rheumatoid factor, but by no means all. It is important, however, that this test is done, as those children who have a positive reading do not have such a good future outlook as those children who do not have this positive finding in their blood.

Pauciarticular juvenile chronic arthritis

This type of arthritis is diagnosed when four, or fewer, joints are involved in the disease process. Over half of the children with juvenile chronic arthritis fall into this group. Symptoms include:

- **pain, redness** and **swelling** of one – or up to four – joints of the body; it is the knees and ankles that are most frequently affected in this subgroup of arthritis;
- children with this type of juvenile arthritis have **none of the generalized effects** seen in the other two subgroups; they remain generally well, with no fever, throughout the course of the illness.

MANAGEMENT

Adequate **rest** is an important factor in the treatment of children with juvenile chronic arthritis. Complete bed rest is only necessary for those children seriously ill with the disease – namely, those children with the serious systemic type or with many painfully affected joints. But all children with the condition will benefit from an adequate night's rest – around 12 hours every night is a good working figure – and if not actually sleeping, at least resting in bed. Then an hour or two's rest in the middle of the day is advisable.

Physiotherapy plays an important part in the treatment of juvenile arthritis. Once the most acutely painful stage of joint involvement is over, an exercise programme tailored to the individual needs of the child should be planned. The aim is twofold:

- to maintain the mobility of the joints;
- to keep up the strength of the muscles around the joints.

Hydrotherapy pools are valuable for these treatments. The warm water makes painful joints easier to move, and also the buoyancy afforded by the water makes exercising muscles less stressful. The aim is to put all joints of the body through a full range of movement every day.

Splinting of joints is also an important part of treatment. During the acutely painful stages of the disease, specially fitted splints should be worn at night to prevent deformity occurring. These will have the added benefit of preventing pain caused when joints are inadvertently moved during sleep. During the day, splints can give relief from pain when worn over joints in constant use – such as, for example, wrists during a school day.

The **drug treatment** of juvenile arthritis is complex and is dependent upon the type and severity of the disease in each individual child. **Aspirin**, or one of the many other non-steroidal drugs, is the first form of drugs to be used. Each individual child will need careful monitoring, both for benefit from the drug and for unwanted side-effects, when any drugs are prescribed.

Second-line drugs include **gold** and **penicillamine** preparations. Again, these must be careful prescribed and monitored by doctors specializing in the treatment of juvenile arthritis.

Finally, **steroid** drugs are used if treatment with the other groups of drugs is not controlling the disease. The decision to use long-term steroids is one that must not be taken lightly, because of the serious side-effects that can result from prolonged use of these drugs. In children, retardation of growth, as a side-effect, is an ever-present worry. Mixtures of all these drugs, tailored to each child's specific needs, can be used.

Local steroid injections into specific joints can give short-term relief and prevent total loss of function in the joint in selected cases.

Schooling can be continued (as in the systemic onset type) once the acute stage of the disease is over. Limitations on physical activities will need to be sorted out between educational and health staff. Generally speaking, competitive sports such as football, hockey and sprinting are not suitable. Even if the child feels able to compete, energies should be tactfully diverted into other activities more suitable for potentially damaged joints. For example, swimming as a sport is one in which the child with juvenile arthritis should be able to keep up with peers. Also, as a leisure activity, cycling is suitable. (It is advisable to be sure that the atlantoaxial joint – at the base of the skull – is stable before commencing any sport.)

For children with severe disease, **special schooling** may be necessary.

Occupational therapists can also provide valuable help for the severely affected child who has difficulty with such everyday activities as dressing, toileting or eating. Much help can also be given to provide suitable activities when long periods of bed rest become necessary for children severely affected by the disease.

COMPLICATIONS

Complications affecting the eye are the only ones in parts of the body other than the joints. Here, a condition known as iridocyclitis can occur. Long-term inflammation of different parts of the eye can lead to cataract formation and/or glaucoma. These later effects are seen more frequently in children having the pauciarticular type of juvenile chronic arthritis. Surgical treatment for cataracts may be necessary at a later date, and glaucoma may need surgical or drug treatment.

Complications can also occur as a result of the necessity of **long-term drug treatment**, especially if the steroid drugs have to be used for any length of time. **Slowing of growth** can occur under these circumstances, together with an increased susceptibility to **infections** of all kinds. **Osteoporosis** (thinning of the bones) can also be a result of the long-term use of steroids – as well as of the disease itself.

THE FUTURE

Juvenile chronic arthritis is a long-term disease, and the future will depend on both the type of disease and the response to treatment. Some children will be severely handicapped throughout life by their arthritis. They may need later surgery to replace disorganized and useless, painful joints or to release tight muscles that are causing deformity. But 70–80% of sufferers will lead useful, independent lives.

In less severe manifestations of the arthritis, adequate splinting during exacerbations of the disease will do much to keep deformity to a minimum. Physiotherapy, on a long-term basis, is also vital to preserve mobility of joints and muscle strength.

SELF-HELP GROUPS

Children's Chronic Arthritis Association
47 Battenhall Avenue
Worcester, WR5 2HN
Tel. 01905 763556.

Lady Hoare Trust for Physically Disabled Children
87 Worship Street
London, EC2A 1BE
Tel. 0171 377 7567.

Young Arthritis Care
18 Stephenson Way
London, NW1 2HD
Tel. 0171 916 1500.

Asthma

Incidence

It is difficult to quote the exact incidence of asthma, partly because of problems with the precise definition of this condition. The interface between 'wheezy' bronchitis and asthma have been blurred, making for difficulties in quantifying the disease.

Recently, figures for school children in the UK with asthma have been quoted to be as high as 1 in 4. A research project has shown that one child in every seven takes an inhaler to school to use if s/he feels an attack of asthma is imminent. So, if the condition is underdiagnosed and treatment other than with inhalers is taken into account, the figure of 25% may not be so far from the truth.

There are other reports pointing to an increasing incidence of asthma, such as:

- 8000 emergency severe asthma admissions every year to hospitals in one region of the UK;
- a figure of 1.7 million children in the UK suffering from some degree of asthma;
- 2000 deaths every year in the UK as a result of asthma – 50 children under the age of 15 years making up this figure.

So it would appear that, as well as being a relatively common condition, asthma is increasing in incidence in the UK. But on the 'up' side, it is thought that half of the children suffering from asthma will stop having attacks when they are adults.

The severity of the asthma varies greatly. This ranges from the child with infrequent attacks and no need to stay away from school to the child who needs an inhaler nearby at all times. This latter child may also need frequent hospital admissions to deal with severe life-threatening attacks.

Boys are affected twice as frequently as girls by this condition. There is also often a strong family history of allergies of one kind or another. It is thought that around half the children suffering from severe asthma have someone else in the family who has either asthma, eczema, hay-fever or some other form of specific allergy.

Asthma seems to be less troublesome during the winter months. It has been found that the highest incidence of hospital admissions with asthma was between May and June and between September and November. These times of the year, of course, relate to the optimum times of allergic substances in nature.

Asthma is known worldwide – only in the rural areas of developing countries is the disease rare. The highest rates of increase are seen in the advanced civilizations of the world. It is this fact that leads to the conclusion that environmental factors have a strong influence on the incidence of asthma.

HISTORY

William Osler, the well-known Canadian physician who was a professor of medicine in Oxford during the last century, considered asthma to be a 'neurotic disorder'. Half a century on, this view had undergone a marked change, with asthma being recognized as a distinct clinical entity and treatment for attacks being routinely prescribed. In the late 1960s, Dr Roger Altounyan, a physician deeply interested in immunology, discovered the action of the drugs that today are used to prevent asthma attacks.

CAUSATION

Both heredity and environment are causative factors in asthma.

Hereditary factors, as mentioned previously, play a part as to whether a child suffers from asthma. Any child whose parents or siblings have one of the atopic allergic problems is more likely to be asthmatic than a child who has no such family history. ('Atopy' can be described as any allergic condition in which specific antibodies are produced in response to a variety of outside stimuli. These include such conditions as hay-fever, eczema, allergic rhinitis and allergic conjunctivitis.)

The **environmental factors** that can be involved in the onset of an attack of asthma are legion. They are usually specific to each sufferer, although frequently more than one substance, or group of substances, can initiate an attack.

Probably one of the commonest allergens (those substances to which a child reacts) is the common **house-dust mite**. These are the minute creatures that inhabit the houses – and especially the beds – of even the cleanest and most hygienic of beings. This probably accounts for the large number of night-time attacks of asthma. (It is now known that the season of late summer/early autumn in the UK is the time when the house-dust mites are at their most numerous. This possibly accounts for the increase in asthma during the months of September to November.)

Dogs, cats, horses and other **furry creatures** affect many children. This effectively precludes them from beneficial contact with domestic pets and other animals.

Feathers in pillows can cause attacks of wheezing in susceptible children.

Smoky atmospheres in houses where adults smoke is also a potent factor in the onset of an asthmatic attack.

External factors such as **pollen** from trees and flowers in springtime can be the triggering factor for many children. Media reports of pollen counts in various parts of the country can alert asthma sufferers to take extra precautionary measures.

Of recent years, **air pollutants** in cities from exhaust fumes of cars and lorries have been postulated as a possible cause for the increase in asthma. It is thought that this form of air pollution does not in itself cause asthma, but enhances the allergic response in susceptible people, including children. Microscopic particles from diesel oil have also been implicated, but this has yet to be clarified.

Infection of the upper respiratory tract by viruses is also implicated in the onset of an attack of asthma. (Infections due to bacteria are not thought to produce such a response.) This causative factor is thought to be of special importance in children who seem very prone to infection of this kind.

Intolerance to certain **foods** has been considered to be a factor. This is difficult to prove either way, conclusively, although some parents are quite certain that some foods – specific to each individual child – will bring on an attack of asthma.

Exercise, particularly in cold air, will tend to exacerbate asthma in some children. If the outside temperature is warm and humid, an attack of asthma is not so likely to occur. The warm, humid atmospheres of swimming baths rarely bring on an attack for this reason.

Psychological factors in some children can be a causative trigger. Excitement or worry can result in an attack. Even laughter can precipitate a short-lived wheezy attack, as can crying.

Quite a category of possible triggering factors to be considered when treatment for an asthmatic child is being considered!

CHARACTERISTICS

In children, asthma as a diagnosis should be considered if:

- **wheezy breathing** is heard under specific, but isolated, conditions, e.g. during the course of a viral respiratory infection; on exercise, especially outside on a cold winter's day; and when the pollen count is high – there are other examples in plenty, each dependent on the individual susceptibility of each child;
- the child has a **cough**, especially if this occurs frequently during the night;
- this night-time cough is associated with **breathlessness**.

On **physical examination** there is often little to be learned from listening to the child's chest, particularly if this is done between the attacks of wheeziness. The main purpose in performing this form of examination is to exclude other reasons for the wheezy attacks, which will give specific findings.

A **diary** kept by the child's mother showing when asthmatic attacks occur in relationship to exercise or exposure to any of the other well-known trigger factors is of great value – both in helping to make the diagnosis and in planning treatment.

In severe, long-standing cases of asthma there can be **poor growth** and **chest deformity**.

It may seem strange that these relatively few features occur with such a common, and potentially serious, condition. This is partly why the diagnosis of asthma can be so difficult. It is of interest to note what exactly is happening in the bronchi of the child with asthma:

- a narrowing of the bronchi by the action of the specific allergen on the tiny muscles in the walls of these structures;
- swelling of the mucosal lining of the bronchi;
- sticky secretions partially blocking the narrowed lumen of the bronchi.

When all these three abnormalities occur together, it is no wonder that the child has difficulty in breathing! The 'breathing out' part of the cycle is the one especially affected during an asthmatic attack.

Investigations

A **chest X-ray** is taken initially. This will not show any changes specific to asthma, but will exclude any other reasons for the child's attacks of wheeziness – such as, for example, something stuck in one of the bronchi. (It is amazing for how long a peanut can remain stuck in a small child's bronchi with only wheezy breathing to announce its presence.)

Readings from a **peak flow meter** are the most helpful investigation. These readings can vary at different times of the day, and also in relationship to physical activities.

Skin tests for allergic substances are of limited value. Any child with any allergic symptoms will probably react to most of the common allergens, such as house mite dust, pollen or animal fur.

Management

This is a specialized subject, and in some parts of the country there are clinics devoted entirely to the management of asthma. Treatment will vary depending on both the frequency and severity of the attacks of asthma.

All parents of children with asthma should endeavour to identify, and remove as far as possible, the **triggering factors** in the household. For example, the **household pet** may have to be found another home if contact with the susceptible child brings on asthma. Measures to reduce the amount of **house dust** are important. 'Damp dusting' can help, as can vacuuming of mattresses in an attempt to get rid of house-dust mite. Synthetic fillings for pillows and cushions should be tried in case the child is allergic to feathers. (As an emergency measure for getting rid of the mite, try popping the pillows and duvets into the freezer for a while. The house dust mite detests the cold!)

Smoking should be strongly discouraged if any family member has asthma. This rule should also apply to visitors to the house.

Sporting activities should not be discouraged. It is better to give the child suitable medication so that s/he can take part in the school activities than to stop him/her taking part. (It can be a difficult balance to maintain between overprotection of the asthmatic child and allowing him/her to run the risk of a severe asthmatic attack. Parents should receive full explanations of their child's disease, along with advice on how to handle everyday activities and events.)

Schooling for asthmatic children should be along as normal lines as possible. Teachers should be aware of the child's respiratory problems and should know what action to take if an asthmatic attack should occur during the school day. Many children will need to take their inhalers – containing the medication that has been prescribed for them individually – to school. Easy, and quick, access to these inhalers is important for children who are too young to manage their medication for themselves.

Psychological factors, such as anxiety and overexcitement, should be reduced to a minimum. (Parents should be aware, however, of youngsters learning how to get their own way by working themselves up to initiate an attack of asthma.)

If there is thought to be any possible food intolerance, the potentially offending foods should be avoided.

Drug treatment

There are three main groups of drugs used in the treatment of asthma.

- **Bronchodilator drugs**. This group of drugs act by relaxing the muscles around the bronchi. It is the constriction of these muscles that causes the bronchi to narrow in response to an allergen in an attack of asthma. The most commonly used drugs in this group are the ones that act on specific muscle receptors, which are known as **beta-agonists**. They can either be taken by mouth, used in an inhaler or used in a nebulizer. The way in which these drugs are taken will depend on the age of the child and the severity of the asthma. They are only available on prescription. (There are other types of bronchodilator drug available, but these can cause problems with side-effects and so are rarely prescribed. Strangely enough, some of these drugs are available for sale in chemists without a prescription. It is very unwise to buy and give these drugs to children. **Always** contact your doctor if your child has a wheezy cough.)
- **Corticosteroid drugs**. These drugs act mainly by their potent anti-inflammatory action. This means that the swelling and mucous secretions in the bronchi as a result of the allergic reaction are both reduced. These drugs can be taken either by mouth or by an inhaler. Side-effects can occur with corticosteroid drugs when taken by mouth if they are used on a long-term basis. One of the most important of

these side-effects to control is the suppression of growth. Serious side-effects do not occur when these drugs are taken by inhaler, although infection with 'thrush' (a fungal infection) can occur in the child's mouth if the inhaler is used over any length of time.

- **Non-steroid drugs** that are used to prevent attacks of asthma. (These were the important drugs discovered by Dr Altounyan in the 1960s.) Sodium cromoglycate is the most frequently used drug in this group, and has revolutionized the treatment for asthma. It is used as an inhaler on a regular basis – usually four times a day – to prevent asthma. It can also be used immediately before undertaking any activity known to precipitate an attack – for example, horse-riding.

The drug treatment of asthma is a complicated one, needing constant review over the years. This is especially necessary for asthmatic children, as the severity and pattern of their asthma can vary throughout the years of growth. Special asthma clinics are the ideal way to monitor the various possible drug regimes.

The treatment of an acute, life-threatening attack of asthma is very specialized. First-aid measures will include the rapid giving of any specifically prescribed medicine, adequate fresh air, putting the child in the most comfortable position (usually sitting forward and leaning on a table) and calling the emergency services on a 999 call. Open access to the ward has proved to be very advantageous for the child with asthma.

Parents should be warned not to overemphasize their child's asthma.

The future

Asthma is a condition that can burn itself out in childhood, so that very few, if any, attacks are suffered in adulthood. This will apply to around half the children who have asthma during their childhood years. It is impossible to predict which child will continue to suffer from asthma throughout life. A strong family history of allergic disease is not an encouraging feature from this point of view.

SELF-HELP GROUPS

National Asthma Campaign
Providence House
Providence Place
London, N1 0NT
Tel. 0171 226 2260
This group has a number of useful leaflets available on all aspects of coping with asthma.

The British Lung Foundation
Kingsmead House
250 King's Road
London, SW3 5UE
Tel. 0171 376 5735
can also give helpful information.

Birthmarks

This is a term that probably should no longer be used, as it implies that these marks are something happening at the time of birth. In reality these skin marks are due to some abnormality in the structure of the skin or the underlying blood vessels. However it will take many years before the term 'birthmark' disappears!

Incidence

The incidence of birthmarks is dependent on the type under discussion. The incidence of some types is not precisely known and only a subjective impression is possible. The majority of children, however, have delicate skins with few marks to mar the surface. When 'birthmarks' do occur, they are immediately recognizable, when other internal problems will go unnoticed.

(It is worth remembering the multitude of functions performed by the skin when considering any abnormalities of this vital structure. It is often not realized how many important aspects of body maintenance and health are controlled by the skin. It:

- covers and protects all the underlying tissues from:
  - external injury;
  - excess ultra-violet light;
  - bacteria and fungi around in the immediate environment;
  - excess fluid loss;
- assists in the regulation of body temperature, by means of the sweat glands situated in its structure;
- acts as a sensory organ of touch;
- acts as a synthesizer of vitamin D from sunlight.

The skin can also be a good indicator of health or disease. Just think of the number of conditions – especially in childhood – which have a rash as part of the disease process. 'Birthmarks' usually affect only a relatively small part of the skin and function is not affected, but the cosmetic appearance, particularly on a baby's skin, can give rise to much concern.)

The following are the commonest types of 'birthmark'.

'Stork bites' – alternative name 'salmon patch'

These are small reddened areas, visible from birth, which are seen most commonly on the back of the neck and on the eyelids. (The position of the ones on the back of the neck give rise to the name – the theory being that the baby was carried in the beak of the stork in this position, so leaving the mark!)

There is no treatment required for these, and the marks will usually fade within the first year of life, although the marks on the back of the neck can persist for longer.

NAEVI

This is a large group of skin blemishes, which can be subdivided into two main groups – those that are black or brown in colour and those that tend to have a reddish coloration and arise as a result of an abnormality in the blood vessels.

Congenital melanocytic naevi (CMN)

This rather complex name means that the naevus is present from birth (congenital) and arises from the pigment cells (the melanocytes) in the skin.)

Incidence
It is thought that around 1.5% of the population have one or more of these naevi somewhere on their body.

Causation
It is possible that this condition is inherited in a dominant fashion – so it is worthwhile enquiring if any other member of the family has similar skin markings.

Characteristics
These naevi are present at birth and can be tiny or large – over 20 cm in diameter. The appearance can be **lobulated** with an irregular edge, and some can become **hairy**. The black or dark-brown colour makes them very noticeable.

Complications
There is debate about whether or not there is a significant risk of these naevi becoming **cancerous** in later life. This rarely occurs during the childhood years, and is more likely to happen to the larger naevi. Any rapid change in size or any redness around the edge of the blemish should alert parents to obtain medical advice.

Management
The way these skin markings are managed is very dependent on their size and the position on the body. Small naevi can easily be removed if they are in a very noticeable situation. Larger naevi are more difficult to remove successfully and **skin grafting** may be necessary. Surgeons with expertise in dealing with these lesions will be needed to give advice on the relative benefits and risks of removal.

Laser treatment can remove the superficial pigmented cells and improve the appearance but will not completely cure the problem.

The future

This type of naevus tends not to grow bigger of itself (unless the rare malignant changes occur, of course). Such naevi do, however, enlarge in proportion to the growth of the child.

Vascular naevi

Vascular naevi are lesions based on an underlying abnormality in the blood vessels. There are two main types:

- **haemangiomas** – alternative name, 'strawberry naevus';
- 'port-wine stains'.

Strawberry naevus

Characteristics

Strawberry naevi are not true 'birthmarks'. They are not usually present at birth, but make their appearance during the first few weeks of life. The naevus begins as a **whitened** area – often on the face – that grows rapidly to become a lobulated **bright-red swelling**. This rapid growth can continue for as long as 6 months, by which time the size can be worryingly large and obvious.

The natural sequence of events is that the size of the lesion – after the period of rapid growth has passed – remains constant for a varying length of time. Then greyish areas appear over the surface and the lesion begins to steadily shrink in size. In 90% of cases the naevus will disappear completely by 9 years of age.

If the naevus is on the baby's face and is growing rapidly, this can cause parents much understandable distress. It seems impossible that this bright red swelling, which so mars their baby's appearance, will ever disappear on its own. It can be helpful to have available 'before and after' photographs of babies with a similar naevus to show parents that it really can happen.

Complications

Occasionally, during the period of rapid growth, **ulceration** of the surface of the naevus can occur. This can become infected, and antibiotics are necessary to prevent later scarring. If the naevus is near the baby's mouth or nose, feeding and/or breathing can be difficult. Under these circumstances expert advice is needed as to how best to deal with the problem.

Management

With a relatively small strawberry naevus that is not in a difficult position, nothing needs to be done except to reassure the parents that this blemish will eventually disappear. Routine **measurements** of the size of the lesion, together with assessment of the size of the greying areas, is a helpful boost to morale during the months and years that the naevus is shrinking. For the very large or rapidly growing marks – or those naevi that have become ulcerated – **steroids** will help to slow the growth, as well as antibiotics to control any infection. When the naevus has reduced in size there may be some loose tissue remaining. This may need **plastic surgery** to obtain a smooth outcome. Laser treatment can also be a useful adjunct in difficult lesions.

Port-wine stain

'Port-wine stain' is the very descriptive name given to a group of naevi that are due to a malformation of the capillaries – the tiny blood vessels linking arteries and veins all over the body.

Incidence
It is thought that about 1 in every 10 000 babies is born with this type of naevus. Both sexes can be affected.

Causation
There may be a genetic factor involved, but this is not certain.

Characteristics
Port-wine stains are present at birth and can occur anywhere on the body, although, unfortunately, it is often the face that is involved. Usually only one side of the face is affected. Unlike strawberry naevi, port-wine stains are **flat** and **do not disappear spontaneously**. They start off as small, pinkish spots of varying size, which coalesce to form what appears to be a sheet of coloured skin. With time this colour changes and becomes a purplish hue.

Complications
Again unlike strawberry naevi, ulceration does not happen in a port-wine stain, although later in life the lesion can become much more raised and lobulated. In a very small number of babies a port-wine stain can be indicative of problems with the blood vessels in other parts of the body. The **Sturge–Weber syndrome** is the most serious example of this.

Management
A number of treatments have been tried over the years. These include **surgery** followed by **skin grafting**, various forms of **radiotherapy, carbon dioxide ice** and **cosmetic coverage**. Latterly, the best results seem to be obtained by the use of **lasers**. This treatment needs to be done in short bursts over a period of time.

The future
Apart from the few babies where there is a serious underlying widespread abnormality of other blood vessels, a port-wine stain will only have cosmetic consequences in later life. Not that these can be trivialized, especially if the sufferer is female and the lesion is an obvious one on the face. Good cosmetic cover for marks on the face and psychological acceptance are mainstays of living with a port-wine stain. Hopefully, treatment with lasers will become more successful and widespread.

(These groups are for all kinds of facial disfigurement.)

Junior Let's Face It
14 Fallowfield
Yateley
Camberley, GU17 7LW
Tel. 01252 879630.

Changing Faces
1/2 Junction Mews
Paddington
London, W2 1PN
Tel. 0171 706 4232.

BRONCHIOLITIS

INCIDENCE

Bronchiolitis is the commonest lower respiratory tract infection in babies under the age of 1 year. The peak age at which this particular infection occurs is 3 months, and most episodes of infection occur during the winter months.

The infection can be severe and around 2% of all babies with this disease will need hospital treatment. In 1993, 44 children died from bronchiolitis. Babies who already have other heart or lung disease, such as, for example, a congenital heart problem or cystic fibrosis, will be the most severely ill with the infection. Also, babies living in families where smoking is common are prone to more attacks of bronchiolitis. Similarly, a family history of asthma, as well as overcrowded living conditions and poverty, predispose infants to recurrent attacks of bronchiolitis. Some authorities consider that babies who subsequently develop asthma, or another allergic condition such as hay-fever or eczema, are the ones most likely to suffer severely from this infection.

Boys seem to be more likely to be affected than girls. This is possibly because of the marginally smaller air-passages in boys.

HISTORY

In a similar manner to the classification of epiglottitis, bronchiolitis was not registered as a separate condition in the OPCS (Office of Population and Census Surveys) tables until 1967. Before this time, a general classification of 'respiratory diseases' was used. Figures show that deaths from bronchiolitis have been steadily decreasing over the past two decades, but nevertheless this infectious condition can still be a worrying one.

CAUSATION

The most common causative organism in bronchiolitis is the **respiratory syncytial virus (RSV)**. This virus causes much misery annually to the population at large, and it is thought that by the age of 1 year around 50% of all babies will have been infected. There are a number of different strains, and an episode of illness due to one strain will not provide immunity against other strains. So repeated infections, with similar symptoms, can occur.

RSV is an especially infectious virus and is passed on readily by droplet infection from the respiratory tract or by hand contact, e.g. after sneezing. So it is important that good hygiene is practised when nursing a baby with bronchiolitis to avoid passing on the infection to other children.

Other viruses can also cause bronchiolitis, but are less commonly implicated than RSV.

CHARACTERISTICS

Bronchiolitis is an inflammation of the tiny air-passages leading to the alveoli of the lungs where the actual gaseous exchange of carbon dioxide and oxygen takes place.

The illness starts in a similar way to a head cold – a **runny nose** and a **fever**. A **cough** develops within 2–3 days and the baby will be heard to **wheeze** as each rapid breath is taken. Breathing will became more rapid, and the area of the body below the ribs will be seen to be sucked in with each breath.

As the infection worsens, **feeding difficulties** can be experienced. These are due to the problems the baby has in co-ordinating swallowing with the rapid difficult breathing. On listening to the chest, **crackles and squeaks** can be heard all over the lungs.

As the disease progresses, the baby can become exhausted with the effort of breathing. **Cyanosis** – a blue coloration of the skin due to lack of oxygen – can also occur in severe cases.

MANAGEMENT

Babies with a mild attack of bronchiolitis can be safely nursed at home. But if the baby becomes:

- **toxic**, with a rise in temperature and breathing rate;
- **exhausted** with the effort of breathing;
- **difficult to feed**;
- **cyanosed**,

hospital treatment will be necessary.

Medical advice is necessary in all but the mildest of infections. Diagnosis and possible subsequent hospital admission is a decision that needs to take into account home circumstances as well as the severity of the infection.

In hospital, continual **monitoring** of the baby's general state will need to be done with adequate **provision of fluids** and feeds. In severe cases **assisted ventilation** of the lungs will need to be done. The baby should be disturbed as little as possible during this time.

Antibiotics play no part in the treatment of this viral infection. It is only if secondary infection with bacteria occurs – as seen by the worsening of the baby's condition with a rise in temperature and an obviously infected nasal discharge – that antibiotics have any effect on the course of the illness.

An antiviral drug has been tried in America, but has been found to be of the greatest use for babies who have bronchiolitis on top of an already severe lung problem, such as cystic fibrosis.

PREVENTION

While there is little that can be done to completely exclude bronchiolitis, the following can reduce the incidence:

- the household in which the baby lives should be a **non-smoking** one;
- **good hygiene practices,** such as hand-washing and control of coughing and sneezing;
- particular care of infants with other **underlying heart or respiratory conditions;**
- early medical involvement for young babies having **feeding difficulties** due to breathing problems.

For many years attempts have been made to produce a **vaccine** against RSV, but so far with no permanent success. However, further preparations are currently being tested.

THE FUTURE

Babies who have had an attack of bronchiolitis often have recurrent 'wheezy' episodes throughout early childhood. A few will subsequently develop asthma.

BRONCHITIS

INCIDENCE

Bronchitis is a common condition, especially during the cold winter months. Much confusion has arisen – and still arises – over the differentiation of 'wheezy bronchitis' and asthma. (This is discussed further in the text under 'asthma'.) Bronchitis is an inflammation of the bronchi – the cartilaginous tubes leading from the trachea (windpipe) to the alveoli of the actual lung tissue. It is in these minute alveoli that the actual gaseous exchanges take place, and when infection reaches this part of the lung, it is known as pneumonia.

While children up to the age of 5 years suffer, on average, from around six upper respiratory tract infections every year, relatively few of them go on to suffer from bronchitis.

Teething and bronchitis together are a well-known facet of folklore. In reality there is no connection between this infection and the entirely normal process of cutting teeth. It is just possible that the pain and upset that some children suffer when their teeth are erupting can lower their resistance to infection. It is perhaps because of this aspect that bronchitis can sometimes occur at the same time as the teething process.

The incidence of bronchitis in older children is variable, a mild attack of bronchitis sometimes occurring with an upper respiratory infection. Those children who have recurrent 'wheezy' bronchitis are probably suffering from asthma.

CAUSATION

Bronchitis usually arises from a viral infection. These infections usually begin in the nose and throat, and then descend, in some children more frequently than others, to the lower respiratory tract. It is less usual for there to be a bacterial cause for bronchitis, although there can be added bacterial infection following on from an initial viral infection.

Measles and whooping-cough – a viral and bacterial infection respectively – are always complicated by bronchitis to some degree.

CHARACTERISTICS

Bronchitis usually follows on from, or is seen in conjunction with, an upper respiratory tract infection – the symptoms of which are well-known to everyone! – a runny nose, sore throat and maybe a mild fever.

The one diagnostic symptom of bronchitis is a **cough**. This cough is dry in the early stages, but within a day or two will become loose, and yellowish **sputum** may be coughed up. Children, however, tend not to cough up secretions but to swallow them. This can on occasions cause **vomiting**.

A **wheeze** can also be heard in some children with bronchitis. This is due to the narrowing of the bronchi as a result of the infection. (The wheeze is caused by the air passing through the narrowed passages.) But this, as mentioned previously, can also be a manifestation of asthma. There may be, but not invariably, a mild **fever**, together with general feelings of **malaise**. The child may also be reluctant to eat.

On listening to the child's chest with a stethoscope, the typical sounds of the air passing through the inflamed bronchi can be heard.

MANAGEMENT

In a straightforward case of bronchitis antibiotics are of no value, as the infection is usually viral in origin. (Antibiotics have no action against viruses.)

A **light diet**, with plenty of **fluids** (of the child's preference) with play in a warm room is all the treatment that is necessary.

If the cough becomes excessively irritant, keeping the child – and the rest of the family – awake at night, a **soothing linctus** can be given. A mixture containing glycerine, honey and lemon is suitable, and can be obtained from chemists. (Other proprietary cough mixtures, many of which have a cough suppressant action, are not advisable. The cough is part of the body's natural defence mechanism, being useful in removing infected material from the lower respiratory tract.)

If the child with bronchitis is particularly wheezy, medication to dilate the bronchi can be prescribed to good effect.

Attendance at school should cease until the worst of the cough has cleared and the child is feeling able to cope with the physical demands of school again.

In an uncomplicated attack of bronchitis the cough will clear within a week to 10 days, and the child will return to full health.

COMPLICATIONS

Secondary bacterial infection of the bronchi can occur. Under these circumstances, the cough will be showing no signs of improvement, and may even be worsening. The child may also become more feverish, or run a fever where there has been none before. Antibiotics will be needed to clear the infection under these conditions.

Pneumonia, where the infection reaches the alveoli of the lung, can be a complication of bronchitis. Again this infection can be due to a either a virus or a bacterium. (Pneumonia can occur, of course, without a preceding upper respiratory tract infection or bronchitis. This is especially the case in premature babies, children who have some congenital defect or those children who are malnourished.)

The infection can affect either the whole of a lung (or both lungs) or a segment or lobe of a lung. The former is known as bronchopneumonia and the latter as segmental or lobar pneumonia.

The child with pneumonia will be seriously ill. There will be a rapid rate of respiration – this is in direct contrast to the picture seen with bronchitis, where the respiratory rate is within normal limits. The child's nostrils will be dilated as s/he struggles to get air into the lungs. The cough will be persistent and irritating, and fever will be high – altogether a far more severe set of symptoms than is seen with an attack of bronchitis.

Investigations if pneumonia is suspected include a chest X-ray, a throat swab and blood test to be examined in the laboratory for the infecting organism.

Hospital admission is necessary for the child severely ill with pneumonia. Nursing in an oxygen tent and intravenous fluids may be necessary during the initial acute stages. Antibiotics are necessary to cure the infection. Even if the initial pneumonia was caused by a virus, secondary infection with bacteria is common.

Older children with a less severe attack of pneumonia can be nursed at home if the home circumstances are suitable. Parents should always be encouraged to contact their doctor again if they are at all worried about their child's condition.

THE FUTURE

Uncomplicated bronchitis will have no permanent after-effects on the child. It is when the symptoms become blurred with those of asthma that long-term effects – due to the asthma – may occur.

Chickenpox

Alternative name

Varicella.

Incidence

The exact incidence of attacks of chickenpox in children is not known. It is, however, a common and highly infectious disease occurring most usually in the 2–8-year age group. Chickenpox is found all over the world except in a few isolated communities. In children the disease is usually a mild one with few complications or permanent after-effects. In adults contracting the disease this picture can be different, serious illness occasionally being the result. So, from this point of view, it is preferable that chickenpox should be contracted during childhood. (Introduction of the infection to isolated communities who do not generally suffer from chickenpox can also be serious.)

There are two groups of children in whom an attack of chickenpox can also have serious results. These are:

- children who are receiving immunosuppressant drugs for some other condition;
- very young babies.

In both these groups chickenpox can be a life-threatening disease. Hospital admission will be necessary.

Causation

Chickenpox is caused by a virus. Immunity, gained by a naturally acquired attack of the disease, is usually lifelong, so that second attacks are extremely rare. But it is not unusual, however, for an attack of shingles to occur in later life, often following a period of general debility. This is due to a reawakening of the virus, which has lain dormant in the body for many years. On the other side of the coin, a child can contract chickenpox from a grandparent with shingles.

Chickenpox has an incubation period of 14–21 days with, most usually, the next member of the family showing signs of the infection on around the 16th day. The infection is most likely to be transmitted during the first few days of symptoms. The virus is then present in the saliva, so that droplet infection from the breath or during sneezing or coughing is the common mode of passage of the virus.

CHARACTERISTICS

The infection starts, in many children, with a mild non-specific illness with a general feeling of **malaise** and frequently a **low-grade fever, headache** and occasionally a **sore throat** – in fact very similar to the symptoms and signs of a common cold. It is not until the appearance of the typical rash that chickenpox can be said to be the cause of the original symptoms.

The rash passes through three stages. Firstly, there is a raised, red, discrete rash which, within a very short time, will become blistery. It is at this stage that the diagnosis of chickenpox will become obvious. After 2 or 3 days, the clear fluid within the vesicle (or 'blister-like' spot) will become cloudy and of a yellowish colour. As the disease progresses, these spots will crust over, leaving a scab which, if scratched off, can leave a permanent white scar.

The rash appears in crops with 2 or 3 days between the appearance of each crop. Because of this 'cropping', the various stages of the rash can be seen at any one time.

The distribution of the rash of chickenpox is also very specific. Initially, the rash is confined to the chest and face regions of the body, with covered areas of the body having more spots than exposed parts. By the third day, the rash spreads to the limbs. In mild cases relatively few spots occur. But in severe cases the rash can be very extensive and even include the palms of the hands and the soles of the feet. In all but the very mildest of attacks, the rash is also found on the mucous membranes of the mouth and ears, and, in the most severe cases, in the eyes and the vagina.

Severe **irritation** is one of the most unpleasant aspects of chickenpox. This symptom makes its appearance soon after the vesicles have started to crust over. Scratching at this time can cause **scarring** to occur or, more seriously, **infection** of the spots with bacteria.

INVESTIGATIONS

As a general rule with an uncomplicated attack of chickenpox no specific investigations are necessary. The diagnosis is made on clinical grounds alone.

The virus can be isolated in the laboratory from the fluid in the vesicles during the first 3 or 4 days of the rash. But this is usually an unnecessary exercise, except in unusual cases where there is some doubt about the diagnosis.

MANAGEMENT

General sympathetic care is all that is needed for a mild, uncomplicated attack of chickenpox. A **light diet** with plenty of cool drinks is sensible during the early stages when the child is feeling generally unwell with a fever. Confinement to bed is unnecessary – quiet play in a warm room is all that is needed.

Calamine lotion and frequent **tepid baths** will do much to allay the irritation of chickenpox. If the itching is a problem in spite of this treatment, an **antihistamine cream** can be tried. Finger-nails should be cut as short as possible to prevent injury through scratching. **Aspirin must never be given to children with chickenpox** because of the link between the use of this analgesic in chickenpox cases and Reye's syndrome.

Schooling can be resumed after 1 week from the onset of the rash if (and only if) the child is feeling perfectly well. Once the spots have crusted over, transmissions of infection is no longer a problem – the scabs contain no active virus. Many children are sent home from school because they still have a few crusted spots. This is an unnecessary precaution from the transmission of infection point of view. It is only if the child is still feeling unwell that s/he should be at home.

Complications are rare with an attack of chickenpox.

- **Secondary infection** of the rash, due to scratching, is the most usual complication of this mainly mild disease of childhood. Antibiotics may be necessary if this is severe.
- **Pneumonia** can occur in adults or immunosuppressed children with an attack of chickenpox. Children without other underlying disease will not suffer from this complication.
- **Encephalitis** is a further possible, but rare, complication.

PREVENTION

There is at present **no immunization** available against chickenpox, although research into this possibility is taking place. With such a generally mild disease of childhood with few serious complications a vaccine for general use would seem to be unnecessary. For immunosuppressed and otherwise ill children, however, the picture is different, and a vaccine to prevent the infection would be of use.

Quarantine measures are unlikely to succeed as chickenpox is such a highly infectious disorder at a time before the diagnosis becomes obvious.

THE FUTURE

There are generally no future problems following an attack of chickenpox. The only possibility is an attack of shingles later in life due to reactivation of the dormant virus.

Coeliac disease

Incidence

Coeliac disease appears to be predominantly a condition seen among people of European and American origin. While it is not unknown in the Far East and Africa, the incidence does not appear to be as high as in America and Europe. This may, however, be due to differences in the recording of disease types. In the UK, the incidence is reported as being between 1 in 2000 and 1 in 6000 – quite a wide variation. (In Northern Ireland, the incidence has been said to be as high as 1 in 300.)

History

This condition was recognized in children over 100 years ago, but it was not until the early 1950s that the relationship between coeliac disease and the eating of wheat-flour products was noticed by a Dr Dicke. Later in the 1950s, the pathological changes in the small intestine were described.

Causation

Coeliac disease is one of the many malabsorption conditions found in both adults and children. There are a great number of these conditions – some mild, some serious, some temporary, some permanent – in which the malabsorption of food is the basic cause. Coeliac disease is one in which there is an allergic response of the small intestine to the substance gluten, to be found in wheat and wheat products. Some sufferers are also allergic to a similar substance to be found in barley, oats and their products.

It is thought that there is a basic immunological fault in the individual with coeliac disease, causing the pathological changes seen in the small intestine following the eating of gluten-containing products. There appears to be a high familial incidence, although no specific genetic link has, as yet, been found.

Characteristics

The age at which an affected child will show signs of coeliac disease varies between 9 and 18 months. The onset follows fairly soon after the beginning of mixed feeding, with the inevitable inclusion in the diet of wheat products.

There are two main ways in which coeliac disease manifests itself.

- There can be a relatively acute onset with **diarrhoea, lack of appetite** and a marked **abdominal distension**. Over the succeeding weeks, there is a loss of weight. In the child with fully developed, untreated coeliac disease, the contrast of the grossly distended tummy with the starkly thin buttocks and thighs is very marked.
- A slower, more insidious onset may occur, with signs of **lack of growth** both in height and weight and the development of an **iron-deficiency anaemia**. (The importance of serial measurements of height and weight, recorded on a centile chart, is highlighted once more in this condition.)

The child with coeliac disease will also tend to be miserable, complain of tummy-ache and generally be off-colour.

INVESTIGATIONS

As well as the clinical and serial measurement signs noted, examination under the microscope of a small piece of the intestine is necessary to confirm the diagnosis. This is known as a **jejunal biopsy** and relates to the specific part of the intestine, the jejunum, that is examined. This process is carried out by the child swallowing a special capsule – the Crosby capsule. This tiny instrument removes a small part of the intestine. The capsule is then recovered later from a bowel motion.

On examination under the microscope, the appearance of the lining of the small intestine is quite unique if coeliac disease is present. The normal picture is of a series of 'ridges' in the membrane. This makes for a large surface area through which absorption of food materials can occur. In coeliac disease these 'ridges' (in adults these structures are more finger-like and are known as 'villi') are completely absent. The result of this is that very little food can be absorbed.

Specific **blood tests** for iron and a specific antibody against gliadin (the protein in the gluten) can help with the diagnosis, as can also measurement of the **fat excreted** in the motions. But these tests are non-specific, and can also be positive in other disease of the small intestine. So it is always advisable to perform a jejunal biopsy before treatment is started. Ideally, a further jejunal biopsy should be done after several months on a gluten-free diet, when the microscopic picture of the small intestine will be seen to have returned to normal.

MANAGEMENT

The treatment for coeliac disease is a **gluten-free diet**. Within a few weeks a vast improvement will be seen in the young sufferer. S/he will begin to gain weight, the diarrhoea (if this has been a problem) will cease, and s/he will have more energy and be altogether a happier, easier-to-manage child.

At first sight the exclusion of all wheat-containing foods from the diet can seem daunting. But with advice from a dietician, and help and encouragement from the Coeliac Society, mothers and child-carers will soon become used to the new regime. In the light of present knowledge, a gluten-free diet should be adhered to for life.

It is vital that the child with coeliac disease should have **regular reviews** to be sure that normal growth and development are being maintained. At these reviews any problems with diet can also be ironed out.

Some authorities advise a **gluten challenge** after 2 or 3 years on the gluten-free diet. Wheat-containing foods are reintroduced into the diet and a further jejunal biopsy is performed. If the appearances under the microscope have regressed to the pre-gluten-free diet again, the diagnosis of coeliac disease is 100% correct. A further reason for performing these serial jejunal biopsies is to be sure that the gluten intolerance is permanent and not a transient phenomenon.

Children in whom the diagnosis has been delayed may need **dietary supplements** of vitamins and minerals for a short time until these important substances are able to be properly absorbed again. Specifically, the absorption of the mineral iron, and vitamins D and K, can be especially affected.

COMPLICATIONS

These are unusual, but if they do occur are readily rectified.

An **iron-deficiency anaemia** can occur in children in whom the diagnosis is delayed or difficult. Iron by mouth or injection will readily cure this.

Rickets due to lack of vitamin D absorption can also occur very occasionally if the diagnosis is delayed for any reason. Here again, vitamin D supplements will halt this process.

During the difficult period of **adolescence** strict adherence to the gluten-free diet may be less than perfect! No adolescent wishes to be eating different foods from their contemporaries and they often rebel against advice. Initially, only minimal effects are seen, but eventually there will be a return of the malabsorption symptoms. Sensitive handling during this period can reduce problems to a minimum. (Perhaps this is hardly a 'complication', but nevertheless it is a situation that frequently occurs and one to be remembered during the adolescent years.)

THE FUTURE

There has been a reported increase in the incidence of intestinal cancer in people with coeliac disease. But this has not been fully elucidated. Also, it is not entirely clear whether strict adherence to a gluten-free diet throughout life has any bearing on this future possibility.

The Coeliac Society
PO Box 220
High Wycombe
Bucks, HP11 2HY
Tel. 01494 437278.

SELF-HELP GROUP

Congenital dislocation of the hip

Incidence

The incidence of congenital dislocation of the hip (CDH) is around 1 in every 1000 births in northern Europe. There is a further group of babies – quoted as being as high as 1% of all births – who have 'unstable' hips, i.e. hips that are potentially capable of becoming dislocated. This latter group of babies need careful follow-up until they are walking satisfactorily.

The incidence of CDH is especially high in Japan and also among peoples who tightly 'swaddle' their babies, such as Lapps and native Americans. The hips of babies who are tightly wrapped, or 'swaddled', remain in an extended, or straight, position for many hours. This means that if there is any underlying instability of the hip, dislocation can occur more readily – as well, of course, as the instability persisting into later childhood.

Girls are affected five times more often than boys. Both hips can be affected or only one. In this latter case, it is more usual for the left hip to be affected.

History

Routine screening of all newborn babies for dislocated hips only began in the 1950s and there is still much to be learned about the incidence and causes of this condition as well any long-term effects in later life.

Causation

It is considered that both genetic and environmental factors can be contributory causes to congenital dislocation of the hip. These different factors will be specific to each individual child.

Direct inheritance seems to play a small part in the causation, although a definite form of dominant inheritance has been reported from one large family who had several members with the problem. It is, however, probable that – as with many other conditions – there can be a familial tendency to abnormalities in the hip joint.

The markedly higher incidence seen in girls may have something to do with the influence of female hormones on the laxity of the ligaments surrounding joints in general and, in this case, the hip joint in particular.

Prenatal factors, such as the baby lying in the breech position for some time, and also, for some obscure reason, a first-born baby, are further potential risk factors.

Characteristics

The hip is a 'ball-and-socket' joint in which the 'ball' of the head of the thigh bone fits neatly into the 'socket' on the pelvic bone.

In the newborn baby a congenitally dislocated hip will not be noticed unless specific screening tests are done to detect the condition. It is only when the child begins to walk that the problem becomes obvious. At this time there will be a **limp,** a very specific **waddling gait,** possible **pain in the hip** and a **reluctance to walk far.** All these signs and symptoms are not necessarily present in each individual child, but any combination of these should alert parents to seek further investigation. Hopefully this situation will never arise if the tests for congenitally dislocated hips are done in the early days of life. These are as follows.

- If only one hip is affected it may be possible to notice in the new-born baby a **shortening** of the affected leg; similarly, at this time a difference in the **position of the folds** in the two legs can be obvious.
- There are two specific manoeuvres that are carried out to detect a dislocation or potential dislocation as in an unstable hip. These tests are termed the **Barlow** and **Ortolani manoeuvres.** They rely on the ability of the examiner to – very gently – test whether or not the head if the femur (the thigh bone) can be moved in and out of its normal position in the pelvic bone. (In no way do these tests hurt the baby or cause distress in any way.)
- These screening tests need to be done three times during the first year of life – in the immediate newborn period, at 6 weeks of age and at around 9 months of age.
- It is of especial importance that tests for CDH are carried out on babies who are at a potentially high risk, such as:
  - babies who have some other family member who has the condition;
  - babies who have been lying in the breech position for some weeks before birth;
  - babies who have some other positional problems, such as talipes (an in-turning of the foot). It is thought that up to 20% of babies with CDH have some other positional difficulties.

Any query as to the stability of the hip – or hips – following these screening tests will need treatment and close follow-up over the succeeding weeks and months. Referral for continuing care by an orthopaedic surgeon is the usual course of action.

Investigations

X-ray examination of the hip is unhelpful as the bones in this area of the baby's body are not as yet ossified so as to be visible on X-ray.

Ultrasound examination is of value and research is continuing into this method of detecting CDH. At present in the UK this method is largely used to assess babies who are found to have an unstable hip on clinical examination, as well as monitoring the success of treatment in babies with a definite dislocation or instability.

It must be emphasized that these screening procedures will not necessarily identify all children with a CDH. So it is of vital importance that parents should report any worries they may have regarding their child's walking abilities – at least until 2 or 3 years of age, when this skill should be fully attained.

MANAGEMENT

The aim of treatment for unstable hips is to keep the head of the femur firmly in the pelvis. This is done by keeping the baby's legs in a frog-like position by means of special **splints** for up to 3 months. This ensures that as growth proceeds, stimulation to the development of the joint is correctly applied. Caring for a baby who is being nursed in one of these splints can cause parents some initial difficulties:

- prams and cots need to be wide enough to accommodate the baby lying in the 'frog' position;
- nappy changing can be more difficult, as can washing;
- rubbing of the splint on delicate skin must also be carefully checked so that pressure sores do not develop.

Special equipment loan facilities are provided locally in the UK for this type of treatment. Advice and literature on caring for babies during this time is also available from self-help groups.

For hips that are completely dislocated, it is necessary to apply gentle **traction** until it is possible to place the hip joint into its correct position. Following this, the splinting process will be necessary to maintain the position.

For dislocated hips that are late in being diagnosed, or those hips that do not respond satisfactorily to splinting, **operation** may be necessary.

THE FUTURE

Early diagnosis and a successful outcome to treatment results in a virtually normal hip joint. Where there is some residual deformity remaining in the joint, degenerative disease with possible osteoarthritis can occur later in life.

SELF-HELP GROUP	STEPS (National association for children with lower limb abnormalities) Lymm Court 11 Eagle Brow Lymm Cheshire, WA13 0LP Tel. 01925 757525.

CONSTIPATION

(Constipation is not a disease entity, but rather a symptom that can be associated with a wide range of conditions. Most frequently, chronic or long-term constipation is the result of an acute event (again due to any number of possible causes) that results in temporary constipation. This symptom is included in the text because of its relatively common occurrence and the concern it can cause both children and their parents. Early diagnosis of the cause followed by appropriate treatment is vital for the well-being of the whole family.)

INCIDENCE

Constipation is not an exciting enough condition for anyone to want to measure the exact incidence. Nevertheless it is unusual for any outpatient paediatric clinic to go by without at least one child being seen for chronic constipation.

Constipation can be defined as delay in the passage of stools, which can reach a chronic state in which the lower bowel is blocked by hard, bulky faeces.

CAUSATION

Causes of constipation are multiple. There are, however, certain groups of conditions that predispose to this symptom.

- There may be some abnormality in the intestine, such as, for example, Hirschsprung's disease (in which there is a much narrowed segment of the intestine) or some gross narrowing around the anal region.
- Conditions in which the child is forced into inactivity because of his/her physical condition can predispose to chronic constipation; examples of this are cerebral palsy, spina bifida and hypothyroidism;
- There may have been an illness in which there has been a high fever. Under these conditions the child can have become dehydrated and/or have eaten little food – both these facts will contribute to constipation which, unless recognized and treated, can become a long-term problem.
- The presence of an anal fissure, in which there is a tiny crack in the skin around the anus, can make defaecation so painful as to put the child off going to the toilet completely! Stools will deliberately be held back. This has the effect of making the faeces hard and bulky and so even more painful to pass. In addition, the lower bowel will

become so stretched that eventually all normal sensation of the need to defaecate will be lost. So a vicious circle is set up.

- Unsympathetic, rigid handling of toilet training in the toddler years can result in the child becoming desperately concerned about this normal bodily function. If this is also followed by inadequate toileting facilities at nursery or school the problem is compounded.
- It is thought that intolerance to certain foods can be a causative factor in the onset of chronic constipation. This fact has always to be considered in a child who also has eczema or asthma.

A sizeable number of problems could thus be causative factors in the onset of long-term constipation.

CHARACTERISTICS

(The characteristics described will be of a long-term constipation and its treatment. The possible underlying causes – outlined above – will also need to be understood and treated.)

The constipated child will often be brought to the surgery with the parents complaining that s/he has **diarrhoea**! This can seem paradoxical, but can be understood when it is remembered that hard faeces are blocking the lower bowel tightly. The fluid waste-products above this blockage will gradually leak and be responsible for soiling the child's underwear, so making the parents think that diarrhoea is the cause of the problem.

On examining the child's abdomen, the hardened faeces can easily be felt. On rectal examination, these solid masses can also easily be felt.

As the problem progresses, so will the urge to have the bowels open diminish because of the overstretching of the lower bowel. This, of course, compounds the problem.

Occasionally the child will complain of abdominal pain when chronically constipated. But surprisingly enough this is not a common complaint.

INVESTIGATIONS

It is not often necessary to do any further investigations other than the initial examination. But occasionally an X-ray of the abdomen will show the extent of the constipation. (This can also be useful in verifying the diagnosis to the parents, who, after all, initially brought their child along with diarrhoea!)

MANAGEMENT

Treatment of any underlying cause for the constipation must be the long-term aim to prevent the condition recurring.

Dietary advice, preferably from a paediatric dietician, regarding adequate fluid and fibre intake is vital.

Treatment of any **anal fissures** with a local anaesthetic cream is also of importance. A good result of emptying the bowel can often be achieved when pain is no longer felt on defaecation. To empty the bowel completely initially, it is usually necessary to give two or more **enemas**. This can be done at the child's home, but it is often more satisfactory to admit the child to hospital for a day or two so that it can be certain that the bowel is completely clear. Following this, a daily dose of a **laxative** should be given to be sure that the bowels are open at least once a day. (A stool softener such as lactulose can be used in conjunction with a stimulant such as senna.) The dosage of the laxative drugs may need to be altered until the right amount is found to produce the desired result without giving the child diarrhoea. This medication will need to be continued until the bowel has been 're-educated'. With the gross overstretching by the hard mass of faeces for some considerable length of time, the child will no longer be aware of the need to visit the lavatory. But as the rectum returns to its normal diameter, normal sensation will return.

Advice on **regular** – relaxed – **times** for visiting the toilet must be given, and practised, alongside the medical treatment. Immediately after breakfast is a good time (if an adequate period of time can be found at this often stressful time of the day). Food in the stomach can initiate the 'gastrocolic' reflex, which helps with bowel elimination.

A system of '**star charts**' can sometimes be helpful (as with enuresis – see elsewhere in the text). The child is encouraged to note on the chart the days when the bowels have been successfully opened. Emphasis must always be placed on success, rather than note taken of failure.

This regimen will have to be continued for some considerable time before full success is achieved – months rather than weeks. Both parent and child can become disheartened by this need for lengthy treatment. So it is important that adequate **support** is given throughout this time by all involved – general practitioners, health visitors, clinic staff and dieticians.

In the event of no – or little – success over a considerable period of time, there may be need for **further investigation** to be sure that there is no anatomical or other abnormality that is giving rise to the chronic constipation.

Also, it is worth checking that the child has no hidden **fears** of visiting the toilet.

THE FUTURE

This is, of course, dependent upon the basic cause of the constipation in childhood. If there is no underlying abnormality, constipation need no longer be a problem in later life as long as a suitable diet and regular bowel movements are made a part of everyday living.

CROUP

INCIDENCE

This upper respiratory condition affects children from the age of 18 months upwards. After 2 years attacks of croup become less common. It is thought that as many as 10 000 children every year in the UK are admitted to hospital with croup – even if only for a short time.

CAUSATION

Both bacteria and viruses can be the causative organisms involved in croup. The most usual bacteria to be involved are the *Streptococcus*, *Staphylococcus* and *Haemophilus influenzae* bacteria. The more usual infections, however, are caused by the parainfluenza virus or respiratory syncytial virus. All these organisms are common causes of recurrent upper respiratory tract infections in children – and adults. This type of croup – due to an infection – is more usual in children over the age of 3 years.

Some allergic children have frequent attacks of croup. These attacks are not thought to be always necessarily associated with an infective process, but rather a hyperactive response in the airways. Younger children are often more susceptible to this type of croup – possibly because of the relatively smaller size of their air passages.

CHARACTERISTICS

Children with an infective type of croup will start with the usual symptoms of a head cold – a **runny nose, poor appetite** and a **fever**. Within 24–48 hours a **barking cough** will follow, and with each indrawn breath there will be a loud, harsh, wheezing noise known as **stridor**. This can be particularly severe at night.

The child will be restless and there can be an **indrawing of the ribs** with each difficult breath – an extremely worrying picture for parents. In severe cases **cyanosis** – a bluish tinge to the skin – can occur. This latter sign is serious and shows that the child's airway is in danger of complete obstruction.

Children with recurrent attacks of croup have no head cold symptoms before the onset of the harsh barking cough. There will be no fever and stridor is less than with an infection. This type of croup is an altogether milder type, but can, of course, progress if added later infection intervenes.

(Other conditions in which stridor is a feature must be excluded. For example, an inhaled peanut or other small object can give rise to a similar noise, and epiglottitis is a possibility in the younger age group that must not be forgotten.)

MANAGEMENT

Children with an infective type of croup will need urgent medical advice, because of the rapidity with which airway obstruction can occur. Depending on the severity, **hospital admission** to a unit where there are facilities available to deal with obstructed airways is often necessary. **Oxygen** can be necessary to aid gaseous exchange in the lungs, and **steroids** can be helpful in reducing symptoms. If the infecting organism is thought to be a bacterium, **antibiotics** will need to be prescribed.

For children with an allergic attack of croup, home remedies, such as nursing in a room with a **steaming kettle**, together with a **mild sedative**, can help. However, these remedies must never delay the calling for medical help if the condition is not improving rapidly or is worsening.

THE FUTURE

Croup usually ceases by the time school days start. Wheeziness, cough and milder attacks of stridor can occur, of course, throughout life. This can be due to both allergic and infective causes – such as asthma and laryngitis, for example.

DEAFNESS

Deafness itself is not a disease entity. It can be a symptom of many types of disorder, ranging from congenital and inherited problems to infections of all kinds and also injuries.

There are two types of deafness – **sensorineural deafness**, in which the actual nerves of hearing are involved, and **conductive deafness**, in which there is interference in the passage of the sound waves to the nerves of hearing. These two types will be dealt with separately as, although the outcome – deafness – is the same, aetiology and treatment differ.

SENSORINEURAL DEAFNESS

Incidence

A sensorineural hearing loss affects around 1 in every 1000 children. This figure includes those children who have a severe hearing loss – in the range 65–80 dB (decibels) – and those with a profound hearing loss – in the range of 85 dB and above.

Causation

There are several possible causative factors for this type of deafness.

- **Genetic deafness** can be inherited in a number of ways, either as a dominant or a recessive characteristic or, in some circumstances, in a sex-linked manner. Certain specific syndromes also have deafness as part of the symptomatology, e.g. Waardenburg's syndrome, Usher's syndrome and Treacher–Collins syndrome. (See Gilbert, P. (1996) A–Z *Reference Book of Syndromes and Inherited Disorders*, Stanley Thornes, Cheltenham, for descriptions of these and other syndromes.)
- **Infective causes** can be infections acquired both prenatally and after birth. Infection during pregnancy with Cytomegalovirus, toxoplasmosis or (probably the best known of all) rubella can cause deafness. If any of these infections are contracted at a critical time in pregnancy, during the development of the organs of hearing, congenital deafness can result. Infections contracted during childhood can also cause deafness as a complication. Examples of such infections include measles, mumps and bacterial meningitis.
- **Problems during the neonatal period** (the first 4 weeks of life), such as jaundice or oxygen lack, can result in sensorineural deafness.
- Certain **drugs** can also be a causative factor. Streptomycin used to be a fairly frequent cause of deafness, and a few antibiotics, given

long-term, must be watched for this side-effect. Drugs given during pregnancy can also be the culprits – thalidomide was the best known. Quinine is also known possibly to have a similar effect.

Characteristics

It is vital that a sensorineural deafness in babies is diagnosed as soon as possible. With a severe sensorineural hearing loss from birth, the child will not be able to develop 'inner language' and so will never be able, in later life, to use language adequately.

Checks on hearing are done routinely in the UK at 7–8 months of age. In some areas of the country, the 'acoustic cradle' is used to check the hearing of all newborn babies. A further check-list has been introduced, in 1988, for parents themselves to check their baby's hearing at regular intervals throughout the early months of life.

It is important that any queries voiced by mothers regarding their baby's hearing should be carefully investigated and followed up. Mothers have an instinctive knowledge of problems before they are fully obvious to other people.

Babies at greater risk of deafness because of a strong **family history** of poor hearing must also be checked carefully.

Vision should be also watched throughout the child's early life in cases where the cause of the deafness is uncertain. Usher's syndrome, in which there are associated visual problems, can be the reason for the deafness, for example.

Management

Once the extent of the hearing loss has been determined, a plan of continuing treatment and education will need to be formulated. For children with a bilateral loss, **amplification** will be necessary to make full use of any residual hearing they may have. Radio transmission aids are the most successful.

Help from the **services for the hearing-impaired** can give much help and advice to minimize the child's handicap. This assistance will need to be continued for many years.

Many children can be happily integrated into **ordinary schools** with this form of help. A few especially handicapped children will need special schooling and/or teaching by 'signing'. (The most appropriate and successful methods for teaching such children is hotly debated in educational circles. It would seem that an amalgam of all possible methods of communication would be the most satisfactory.)

Any **associated handicap** – such as, for example, the later visual problems seen in Usher's syndrome – must be assessed and managed appropriately.

With specialized – and early – teaching, children deaf from birth can develop understandable speech. The importance of early intervention cannot be stressed too highly.

The future

Career choices must, of necessity, be severely curtailed for children with profound sensorineural hearing loss. Good careers advice should be available from the early teenage years onward.

Later, when a **pregnancy** is contemplated, genetic counselling should be available for the prospective parents.

CONDUCTIVE DEAFNESS

Incidence

This is by far the commonest cause of deafness in children. It is thought to affect around one-third of all children at one time or another between the ages of 2 and 5 years. Although many of these will improve within a few months, up to one-fifth of the affected children will have a hearing loss that persists into late childhood. Both boys and girls are affected.

Causation

The most usual cause of conductive deafness is secretory otitis media. This can occur following an acute attack of middle ear infection. In this condition, sticky fluid fills the cavity of the middle ear, which contains three tiny bones intimately concerned with the hearing process. (Secretory otitis media is frequently referred to as 'glue ear' because of the glue-like nature of the fluid in the middle ear.) Because of this fluid, the ossicles in the middle ear are unable to work adequately. As a result of this, the movements of the tympanic membrane (the eardrum) are restricted, so dulling hearing.

The reason why this fluid persists in the middle ear following an attack of acute otitis media is thought to be lack of drainage of fluid away from the middle ear. Normally, secretions are drained away from the middle ear into the back of the throat via a tiny tube – the eustachian tube. Following an infection, this tube becomes blocked either as a result of swelling of the tissues or by mucus. Young children are especially prone to this, partly because of the relative frequency of upper respiratory tract infections and partly because of the small bore of the eustachian tube in this age group.

Characteristics

The child with a chronic secretory otitis media will often have a deafness of around 20–40 dB. This loss, however, may not be consistent, but fluctuating from week to week. This fact can easily mislead parents into thinking that their child is just 'not attending' during the periods when hearing is less than perfect. Even routine hearing tests may, at times, fail to pick up the hearing loss if the test is performed on a good day.

But even this relatively mild degree of hearing loss can interfere with the **acquisition of speech** in the younger age groups. Speech is learned by imitation of sounds heard. So if some specific frequencies are missed by the child – because of the hearing loss – fully comprehensive speech is attained with difficulty.

In the older child, who has just started school, for example, **behaviour problems** or periods of 'switching off' can occur. Problems such as these can result from the failure to hear instructions adequately – the child compensating in other ways for the failure in hearing. ('Switching off' for short periods can easily be confused with petit mal (see Epilepsy) unless the possibility of a hearing loss is remembered and checked on.

Children with a conductive deafness can also be thought to be **slow learners** if the hearing problem is not recognized and treated appropriately.

Investigations

Clinical examination of the ears of a child suspected of being deaf as a result of secretory otitis media can show a range of abnormalities on the eardrum. The drum can be seen to be pulled inwards and/or of an unusual, greyish colour. There may also be dilated blood vessels coursing across it. The advice of an ear, nose and throat surgeon will be needed in certain children with a view to further treatment.

Audiology tests, suitable to the age of the child, will give information as to the degree of the hearing loss. Under the age of 3 years distraction tests will be needed. After this age most children will be able to cope with pure-tone audiometric tests.

Impedance audiometry can also be used, in especially difficult problems, to determine hearing loss. (This test measures the minute movements of the eardrum in response to sound by means of a special instrument held against the eardrum.)

Management

The best way to treat secretory otitis media that is causing a conductive deafness is controversial. The type of treatment an individual child will receive will depend on the views current in each part of the country. There are three main ways in which the child's hearing can be improved.

- **Antihistamine drugs**, given by mouth, were previously thought to help reduce swelling around the eustachian tube and hence improve the drainage of the middle ear. Along with this treatment, decongestant nasal drops were prescribed for the same purpose. Latter-day thinking is that this form of treatment is of little value.
- An operative procedure – a **myringotomy** – can be performed. In this procedure, the eardrum is pierced (under a general anaesthetic) and the sticky fluid is withdrawn. In addition to the removal of this fluid, tiny ventilation tubes ('grommets') are inserted through the eardrum and left in position. The purpose of these is to ventilate the eardrum in an endeavour to prevent further build-up of fluid. These tubes remain in position for around 1 year to 18 months, when, in the vast majority of cases, they fall out spontaneously.
- **Removal of the adenoids** is also advised by some ear, nose and throat surgeons in an attempt to ease the passage of fluid down the eustachian tube – but again this is controversial.

- Lately, improving the child's hearing with the help of **hearing aids** for a short while is being tried. Results are promising, the children tolerating the hearing aids well.

Most children who have suffered from secretory otitis media with an associated deafness have normal hearing by the time they are 7 or 8 years old. This appears to be the natural history of the disease and is apparently unrelated to the type of treatment previously given. At this time, with this satisfactory result, hearing aids will no longer be required.

One further cause of conductive deafness is a **build-up of wax** in the external auditory meatus – the passage from the exterior down to the ear-drum. This can easily be seen with an auroscope and removed, either by syringing or by making the hard wax more fluid with ear drops. Occasionally it is necessary to soften especially hard wax with ear drops before syringing.

The future

There is rarely any return of the conductive deafness in later life. The usual, temporary, catarrhal deafness following a head cold will, of course, still occur, but rarely persists for any length of time.

SELF-HELP GROUP

The National Deaf Children's Society
15 Dufferin Street
London, EC1Y 8UR
Tel. 0171 250 0123
Fax 0171 251 5020.
This group gives advice to parents on health and education issues, and support through local groups. There are also a number of leaflets available on many aspects of deafness, together with a quarterly magazine.

DIABETES

ALTERNATIVE NAMES

'Sugar' diabetes; diabetes mellitus (the correct name for this condition, which distinguishes it from diabetes insipidus – a condition associated with disease of the pituitary gland).

INCIDENCE

Diabetes is known worldwide and among all races – with a higher incidence among white races. The incidence varies widely. Epidemiology of this disease has unearthed some fascinating facts. It would seem that parts of the world furthest away from the equator (either north or south) have an higher incidence of diabetes than those countries nearer the equator. For example, the number of people with this disease in France is far lower than in Finland. Even such short distances as between the south of England and the north of Scotland show a distinct difference – the incidence being twice as high in Scotland.

The average number of school children with diabetes in the UK is thought to be between 1 and 2 children in every 1000. Diabetes is rare in under-2-year-olds. Adolescence is the most usual time for the onset of diabetes, and in this age group there is a slight preponderance of boys with the condition.

There are two main types of diabetes – the **non-insulin-dependent type** and the **insulin-dependent type**. Children predominantly have the insulin-dependent type, although the other type is not completely unknown. Further discussion will relate to the insulin-dependent type in children.

HISTORY

Diabetes has been known as a disease entity since 1500 BC. It was in the second century that a Turkish physician coined the name 'diabetes' (meaning 'a siphon'). At this time the disease was thought to be a condition arising in the kidneys due to the large amounts of urine passed in the acute disease. It was not until the 19th century that diabetes was known to be a condition caused by malfunction of the pancreas. Dietary measures were the sole treatment available at this time. In 1922, Drs Banting and Best discovered that insulin could be used to successfully treat diabetes. H. G. Wells was a well-known literary sufferer from diabetes. He, and Dr Lawrence, were instrumental in founding the British Diabetic Association.

CAUSATION

Diabetes is due to special cells – to be found in the islets of Langerhans – failing to produce insulin in adequate amounts. Insulin is a substance that is vital to the proper metabolism of sugars in the body. It is this incomplete – or inadequate – metabolism of sugars that gives rise to the symptoms of diabetes.

The precise mechanism of why diabetes occurs is not completely understood. But there are three distinct groups of factors that have a bearing on the onset of the disease.

- **Genetic.** While diabetes is not a truly inherited disease, there are strong family links in the incidence. This is especially so for the insulin-dependent type of diabetes most usually seen in children. Children with two diabetic parents run a greater risk of developing the disease than children who have either only one parent with the disease or no positive family history of the condition. A child with two diabetic parents and a brother or sister with the disease stands a 50% chance of also suffering from diabetes. Recent genetic studies have shown a strong association between the development of diabetes in childhood and a particular 'marker' on chromosome 6. Factors other than genetic ones will then determine whether or not the full-blown disease occurs.
- **Environmental causes** appear to exert some effect on the onset of diabetes. These causes only appear to affect people who already have some genetic predisposition. The commonest of these environmental causes is infection of one kind or another. A viral infection with the Coxsackie B or mumps virus seems especially likely to be a predisposing factor. As most of these types of infections occur during the autumn and winter months, this would relate to the higher incidence during these times of the year. Other environmental factors, such as chemical toxins and nutritional aspects, may also have a bearing on the onset of diabetes in people with a predisposition.
- **Immune mechanisms** have received much interest in later years as possible causative factors in the onset of diabetes. It is known that there is a strong association between insulin-dependent diabetes and autoimmune disease of the endocrine glands such as the thyroid and adrenal glands. Further research into this aspect has important implications for both prevention and treatment of diabetes.

Diabetes is a wide-ranging disorder with many factors to be taken into account when the causation is debated. All people with diabetes probably have a genetic predisposition (known or unknown in the family tree).

CHARACTERISTICS

Diabetes in 90% of children with the disease has an acute onset – usually with a history of various signs and symptoms of less than a month. In the remaining 10%, the same symptoms occur, but in a milder form over a longer period of time.

Symptoms and signs of diabetes in a child include:

- **frequent passage of urine**: this may show itself in some children as a return to bed-wetting (or even daytime wetting) after a period of complete bladder control (it is therefore vital that all children with enuresis should have the urine tested for glucose – see below);
- an **increasing thirst**: as the frequency of the passage of urine increases, so will the child's thirst increase;
- **weight loss**: this loss can occur rapidly in an acute onset of diabetes – the child losing many grams in a week or two;
- **loss of energy**, together with lethargy and exhaustion, will soon become obvious: at this stage the child is seriously ill;
- **irritation** around the vulval region in girls or the penis in boys can occur due to the passage of sugar-loaded urine;
- occasionally **abdominal pain** and **vomiting** may be added symptoms: under these circumstances diagnosis can be delayed if a sample of urine is not tested for glucose – the pain and sickness being thought to be due to a gastrointestinal upset; this type of onset occurs more often in younger children;
- in a severe case of diabetes, the **breath will have a distinctive sweet smell**, similar to that of acetone or pear-drops;
- in a serious undiagnosed case the result can be **coma and death** unless correct and immediate treatment is given.

INVESTIGATIONS

Urine testing for glucose is vital for the early diagnosis of diabetes. If glycosuria is found, there should be an immediate referral to hospital. In a severe case, the urine will also show a positive result when tested for ketones. These substances will be being secreted because of the breakdown of bodily tissues. These chemicals account for the sweet smell on the breath of an undiagnosed diabetic.

Blood tests for glucose will confirm a high level of sugar in the blood. Levels of this blood sugar will need to be done frequently during the subsequent treatment of diabetes.

MANAGEMENT

Treatment for the **acute onset** of diabetes is an emergency. Rapid **hospital admission** is necessary for treatment of the seriously ill child. **Intravenous fluids** and **insulin** are the basis of this very specialized treatment regimen.

A child with a slower and **less acute onset** will still need to be admitted to hospital once the diagnosis is made in order to set up the regimen for the future treatment of the diabetes. (In a very few centres – Leicester in the UK and Tel Aviv in Israel – sufficient expertise is available in the community to treat children at this stage of their illness at home. Continuous ongoing monitoring is vital during these first few days following diagnosis. Usually in these centres this is provided by specially trained nurses.)

About 1 week in hospital is usually necessary to stabilize the diabetes on the dosage of insulin necessary for his/her needs. Much care needs to be taken to be sure that the parents fully understand the basic principles behind the twin methods of the control of their child's diabetes – **diet** and **insulin**.

Diet

For good control of the diabetes, the diet must be tailored to meet the needs of each individual child without causing too much difficulty in adhering to the new pattern of eating. It is necessary to avoid the child feeling unusual among his/her peers, as failure to understand this will cause problems with sticking to the diet.

It is the intake of carbohydrate-containing foods that needs to be controlled in a diabetic diet. Regular measured amounts of this type of food must be eaten. This basically means a helping of carbohydrate: at breakfast; as a mid-morning snack; at lunch-time; as a mid-afternoon snack; at supper; and as a snack at bedtime.

A system of 'exchange' foods is worked out, each unit of 'exchange' food being equal to 10 g of carbohydrate. This system allows for a wide variety of foods to be included, so ensuring that a balanced diet is eaten. The carbohydrate portion of the diet should consist of starchy, high-fibre foods rather than the more quickly absorbed refined sugary foods. These starchy foods are absorbed more slowly over a longer period of time, so giving better control of the diabetes. Such foods include wholemeal bread and cereals, leguminous and green vegetables and fruit of all kinds.

The amount of carbohydrate taken in any one day should be – as a rough guide – 100 g for a 1-year-old child plus an extra 10 g daily for each added year. So, for example, a 10-year-old child will need 190 g of carbohydrate every day.

Each individual child will need to have a daily diet worked out initially by a dietician, together with a list of 'exchangeable' foods. It is surprising how quickly both children and parents become adept at estimating the correct amount of carbohydrate foods that make up a 10 g portion.

Adolescence is a particular time when dietary control can cause problems. Adolescents are not the most sensible of eaters at the best of times, and diabetic youngsters are no exception. Add to these problems the stress of examinations, career choices and boy/girlfriend problems and this time of life can be seen to be fraught with difficulties of control. At this time, too, the child will be moving on from the paediatric diabetic clinic to the adult diabetic clinic. All these changes need sensitive handling.

Insulin treatment

Insulin is needed for the control of the vast majority of diabetic children. Control with diet alone is very rarely achievable in childhood.

The ideal to achieve is to aim to give a regimen of insulin that matches the output of insulin in a normal child. This is virtually impossible to achieve, but every individual child must be balanced on the dose of insulin that matches his/her physiology as closely as possible.

Insulin usually needs to be injected twice a day, although some children may be able to manage on just one daily injection. There are available short-, intermediate- and long-acting insulins, which can be 'mixed and matched' to suit the child's individual needs. This dosage will need to be carefully monitored by the diabetic clinic once the child has left hospital.

During the initial stay in hospital, both parents and child must be fully informed about the nature of the disease and its control. The actual physical process of injecting the insulin must also be taught. Most children over the age of 8 or 9 years will eventually be able to give their own injections, but parents must always keep a watchful eye that this is done regularly and competently.

General management

The child's **school** must be informed of the child's diabetes. Teachers should also be told of the action to take if a hypoglycaemic attack (see below) should occur in school. Such individual needs as, for example, the giving of some readily absorbed glucose before a period of strenuous activity must be fully understood – and implemented – by the staff.

Emotional support will be needed in the early days following diagnosis, especially if the child is the first member of the family to suffer from the disease. Parents must understand that diabetes is a lifelong condition for which, at present, there is no cure. They must equally understand that a full, exciting life can still be led by their child if control of the diabetes is strictly maintained.

Careers for children with diabetes will need to be carefully chosen. The risk of hypoglycaemic attacks in insulin-dependent diabetes is a very real one, and diabetic people are not usually accepted for the armed forces, police or fire brigade because of this. Individual employers usually have their own rules regarding the type of work most suitable for diabetics within their own organizations.

Hobbies, too, will need to be more carefully chosen than for the non-diabetic child. Any activity in which hypoglycaemia could put the child or his/her companions at risk should not be recommended.

Travel may present problems in control. For example, time changes when travelling long distances can cause difficulties in the timing of injections. More – or less – activity on holidays can also make differences in the dosage of insulin necessary.

When the child reaches the age of **learning to drive**, the Driver and Vehicle Licensing Authority, in the UK, must be informed of the diabetic condition. Driving licences are granted on a 3-yearly basis and will need a satisfactory medical report before being reissued. There is rarely any problem with this. (All drivers should, of course, have a supply of sugar in the car at all times to counteract any hypoglycaemia.)

COMPLICATIONS

Hypoglycaemia

Hypoglycaemia (low blood sugar) is an ever-present complication for any-one on regular insulin. As a result of a variety of factors (too little breakfast after having an insulin injection, or too much exercise combined with in-sufficient food, to quote just two examples) the ratio of insulin to carbo-hydrate is upset. Too much insulin or too little carbohydrate will mean that the blood sugar becomes too low and this will give rise to certain specific symptoms:

- dizziness and faintness;
- nausea;
- headache;
- irritability;
- and eventually unconsciousness.

The younger child will be unable to verbalize exactly just how s/he is feeling, and may just say s/he feels 'odd' or 'funny'. Parents and teachers will get to know what is the matter under these circumstances and give ap-propriate treatment. Obviously if the child has become unconscious, a 999 call will be necessary.

Treatment is quick and easy in the early stages of a hypoglycaemic attack. A sweetened drink or a lump of sugar will return the child to normal.

Most hospitals will allow a child to become hypoglycaemic deliberately while the parents are present so that the symptoms can be recognized – and so dealt with quickly.

Later complications

Vision can be affected by diabetes, because of the effect the disease has on the small blood vessels of the body.

As a result of a similar effect on blood vessels the **kidneys** can also be affected, as can other parts of the vascular system.

These latter complications are rarely seen in childhood. Nevertheless it is of importance that good control of the disease is maintained throughout childhood in order to keep these later complications to a minimum.

Special care needs to be taken during **pregnancy** with the control of the mother's diabetes. The baby will also need extra supervision after birth.

THE FUTURE

Diabetes is a lifelong disease and at present can only be controlled and not cured. Research is proceeding along a number of lines, such as a search for possible preventable environmental triggers, the newer types of insulin and the introduction of less toxic immunosuppressant drugs that will allow pancreatic – or islet cell – transplantation.

British Diabetic Association
10 Queen Anne Street
London, W1M 0BD
Tel. 0171 323 1531
      0171 636 6112 (care line).
This group has much useful literature available, together with a diet information service and educational and activity holidays arranged. Research into diabetes is also promoted and funded.

DIPHTHERIA

INCIDENCE

Diphtheria has been an almost unknown infection in western countries for several decades. With the advent of routine immunization of all children against this infection from the late 1940s, the incidence has fallen dramatically. From a figure of around 45 000 a year, with over 2000 deaths, in the late 1940s, the number of cases of diphtheria between the years 1986 and 1991 was 13, with no deaths.

The picture is different, however, in many other countries of the world. In developing countries, diphtheria still takes a tragic toll of young life in terms of both illness and death. However, within the last year or so, there have also been reports of many thousands of cases of diphtheria in Russia and eastern European countries. This emphasizes that continual vigilance is still necessary for the control of this infection.

HISTORY

1881 was the year when the bacteria causing diphtheria was discovered by Dr Theodor Klebs. Soon after this date the toxin produced by the bacteria was described, and in 1894 an antiserum was developed. A further 20 years saw the advent of a preparation that could be used to actively immunize against the infection.

Dr Schick developed, in 1913, a specific skin test by which individuals immune to the effects of the bacteria could be recognized. This test is rarely used today, but, at times can still be of value in determining the immune state of people working in occupations where they might come into contact with the diphtheria bacillus in the course of their work.

CAUSATION

Diphtheria is caused by a bacterium. There are three different strains of this bacterium, giving rise to illness of differing severity. The diphtheria bacillus produces a powerful toxin, which is the cause of many of the generalized symptoms of the illness. It is also this toxin that is responsible for the serious effects seen in the heart and the nervous system.

Diphtheria is spread from person to person by droplet infection, or from clothing contaminated by the organism. Although readily destroyed by heat and antiseptic preparations, the diphtheria bacterium can survive for several weeks in both milk and water. A further way of spread of this organism is from the 'carrier' state, in which some healthy people harbour the organism with no ill-effects themselves.

The incubation period of the disease is between 2 and 7 days.

CHARACTERISTICS

The severity of the infection depends on the strain of the infecting organism – the 'gravis' strain producing the most severe symptoms. At times the infection can be so mild as to pass undiagnosed – the symptoms being thought to be a relatively mild respiratory infection. This, of course, poses problems relating to the spread of the disease – especially among unimmunized children.

In more severe cases the infection will begin with generalized symptoms of:

- **fever**: this does not usually reach as high a level as with a throat infection with the *Streptococcus* bacterium, but can reach 39.5°C; it is important that the two infections are differentiated;
- **headache and general malaise**;
- **sore throat**: this is not such an overwhelmingly unpleasant symptom as the sore throat found in an infection with the *Streptococcus* bacteria, but nevertheless not comfortable. It is later in the course of the illness that the diphtheritic **membrane** appears in some part of the throat. This is a greyish membrane adherent to the underlying tissues which, on removal, leaves the undersurface raw. The danger of this membrane is that it can spread over the whole throat and soft palate – and maybe further down the respiratory tree into the larynx and bronchi – and effectively exclude the passage of air to the lungs.

As the disease progresses, with the production of the specific toxin, the child's general condition deteriorates. The heart muscle can become involved, giving rise to a **weak, irregular pulse**. The **blood pressure will fall** and the child will be gravely ill. In addition, the nervous system can become involved. (These latter serious effects will be seen in an infection with the most serious strain of the diphtheria bacillus in a child who is not immunized against the disease.)

INVESTIGATIONS

Throat swabs – if possible taken from beneath the membrane – will confirm (or otherwise) the diagnosis of diphtheria.

MANAGEMENT

It is vital that **antitoxin** – by injection – is given as soon as possible, before the toxin has become fixed in the tissues. Once this has occurred, the opportunity to counteract its effects is lost. With the giving of antitoxin on the first day of the illness, full recovery is the usual result.

Antibiotics – penicillin or erythromycin – will also be necessary to ensure that a 'carrier' state does not result.

Tracheotomy may be necessary in severe cases where the diphtheritic membrane is causing obstruction to breathing.

Skilled **nursing care** in hospital is necessary for children with a severe infection of diphtheria. (It is also important to remember that added complications – see below – in the heart and nervous system can occur some weeks after the initial symptoms of diphtheria are obvious.)

COMPLICATIONS

Heart. This vital organ can be affected by the toxin produced by the diphtheria bacillus. The heart muscle itself is weakened, and so is unable to perform adequately its function of pumping the blood around the body. It is this direct effect on the heart muscle that causes the irregular heart beat, weak pulse, low blood pressure and other symptoms of heart failure in a severe case of diphtheria.

Respiration can be severely affected if the membrane extends down into the larynx. If this occurs, the sufferer will have a hoarse voice and a 'brassy' cough. Breathing will be extremely difficult and the child will be restless and anxious.

Secondary infection of the respiratory tract by other organisms can occur, giving rise to **bronchopneumonia**.

The nervous system can also be affected by the diphtheria bacteria. Weakness and/or paralysis of any muscle, or group of muscles, of the body can occur. For example the muscles of the eye can be involved, giving rise to a squint, or arms or legs can become paralysed.

These effects occur late in the illness – often many weeks after the involvement of the throat.

PREVENTION

Diphtheria is entirely preventable by immunization, as is verified by the dramatic fall in the incidence of the disease following mass immunization.

In western countries immunization against diphtheria is a stable part of the routine babyhood immunization schedules. In the UK, diphtheria immunization is part of the **'triple' vaccine** offered for all babies at 2, 3 and 4 months of age. A booster dose is given at school entry.

Children who are known to have been in close contact with a case of diphtheria should receive a further injection of vaccine. Close family contacts should also be given a 7-day course of erythromycin to ensure that a 'carrier' state does not result.

THE FUTURE

With early adequate treatment, there are no subsequent effects following an attack of diphtheria – once, of course, the period of time for the late manifestations of the disease has passed. It is if the toxin has severely damaged the heart muscle that late effects in this system of the body can be seen.

ECZEMA

ALTERNATIVE NAMES

Atopic dermatitis; infantile eczema.

INCIDENCE

There are a number of types of eczema, with a variation in classification. **Contact eczema** or **dermatitis** is a good example of an eczematous condition in which there is a definite correlation between the cause and subsequent effect. An example of this is the eczema which can occur in some people on contact with certain metals – the nickel used in jewellery, scissors or cooking utensils – or the rubber preservative chemicals used in rubber gloves.

Eczema affects around 5% of people, and the vast majority of these show signs of the condition in childhood – often below the age of 6 months. Boys and girls are equally liable to be affected.

Hay-fever, asthma and eczema are allergic conditions that frequently occur in different members of the same family. Some 70% of children with eczema have other family members with one or other of these allergic manifestations.

Atopic eczema – the type of eczema that will be further discussed – is a genetically determined skin condition in which specific antibodies can be demonstrated in the blood. Often the 'triggering' factor initiating the rash proves difficult, or impossible, to find.

HISTORY

Eczema has been known since antiquity. The word 'eczema' is derived from the Greek word meaning 'to boil out' – a good descriptive term for the red, bubbling nature of the rash of eczema.

CAUSATION

Genetic factors are certainly at work in the child with atopic eczema, and it may be possible to discover certain foods or conditions that make the rash worse. For example, some babies have an allergy, often temporary, to cow's milk or they are allergic to some particular material found in clothing – wool often being a culprit here. These triggering factors have to be found out by trial and error.

CHARACTERISTICS

The baby/child with eczema will usually have a **dry skin**, which will be in evidence from the earliest days of life.

The typical **rash** of eczema – patches of reddened skin with small blistery spots – is extremely **irritating**. The baby will scratch, making the skin further inflamed and the discomfort even worse.

Eczema typically occurs on the baby's **face** and in the **knee and elbow creases**. In severe cases much of the body can be covered with the rash.

Some children experience a worsening of their rash during **cold weather**, while other sufferers find the rash worst during **hot, humid conditions**. This variability in manifestations of the rash can make management difficult. Each child has to be treated individually.

Improvement in the rash is occasionally seen in children between the ages of 2 and 4 years. Unfortunately, this remission of symptoms is often short-lived, and the eczema returns again during the school-age years.

MANAGEMENT

Children with eczema have – and always will have – a very dry skin. **Emollient (greasy) creams**, applied twice every day, reduce this dryness and minimize the outbreaks of severe eczema. When the worst of the rash is absent, it is important to continue with creams to reduce the dryness.

Soap and bubble bath have the effect of drying the skin even further, and so **should be avoided** for children with a dry skin. Bath oil should be substituted for other bath-time additives, and a minimum of – preferably unperfumed – soap should be used. Moisturizers should always be applied after a bath.

Wool is a particularly frequent irritant to children with atopic eczema. (The distinction here between atopic and contact eczema is blurred.) Most eczema sufferers will react badly to even a minimum of wool in their clothing. Sometimes **acrylic** cloth can also have a deleterious effects. Cotton and cotton/polyester fabrics are the most suitable ones to be worn next to the skin in eczema sufferers. (It must also be remembered that carpets and other furnishing materials can contain a certain percentage of wool. Crawling babies with an eczematous tendency can suffer from the effects of such household furnishings.)

In comparatively rare circumstances, certain **foods** can cause a worsening of eczema. This must be distinguished from the rapid allergic reaction, known as urticaria, which arises when the specific food touches the child's mouth.

Avoidance of any of the above factors which have been shown to worsen the eczema are important in the ongoing care of a child with eczema. Treatment of an acute relapse includes the following.

- A **steroid cream**, applied only to the parts of the skin that have eczematous patches, will help all but the most resistant eczema. These creams should be applied three times daily for a short time. Parents can become concerned regarding the use of steroid creams on their children's skins. They can be reassured that there is no danger of overuse as long as the treatment is not continued for an indefinite period.

- In very severe cases, particularly in young babies where control of scratching is a major problem, **wet dressings** are of value. A greasy cream is applied all over the child's body, with a steroid cream applied to the worst of the eczematous patches. Damped cotton material is then bandaged on over these creams. This treatment needs to be done three times daily, and may need a short stay in hospital. This treatment has the effect of moisturizing the skin which aids the action of the steroid creams. The irritation is reduced and, being completely bandaged, the baby cannot get at the rash to scratch his/her skin.
- If the eczema has become **infected** through repeated scratching, **antibiotics** by mouth will be needed to control this. An antibiotic/steroid cream can also usefully be applied to the rash.
- **Sedation** at night – when the irritation is often at its worst – with an **antihistamine** can also help to reduce the amount of excoriation of the skin.

Eczema is a miserable, long-term problem. Parents and children will need much **support** (preferably from the same doctor, who knows the ups-and-downs of the individual child's eczema) to cope with the inevitable relapses that occur. It is important to emphasise that acute flare-ups can be reduced to a minimum by constant adherence to methods of reducing the dryness of the child's skin and avoidance of known triggering factors.

School days can be unhappy for eczema sufferers if teachers and pupils are not informed of the recurrent and, of particular importance, the non-infectious nature of the condition. There is no sadder sight than a child with eczema being left out of activities because of an exacerbation of the rash and the lack of understanding of his/her peers.

THE FUTURE

Eczema will be a constant companion to many of the childhood sufferers throughout life. When the time comes to choose a career, attention must be paid to avoiding choices that could worsen the possibility of an acute exacerbation of the eczema. Work with chemicals of any kind should be avoided, for example, and hairdressing, where there is much contact with soap products and various chemicals, is not a sensible choice.

SIMILAR SKIN RASHES

There are a number of other forms of skin rash very similar to eczema that are worthy of mention, as confusion is common.

- **Discoid eczema.** As the name implies, this is a true form of eczema, but appears in very specific round patches. In younger children the upper arms and shoulders are the most frequently affected parts of the body. These patches can become very large, with a moist surface. They can be difficult at times to distinguish from impetigo. Steroid creams and moisturizing ointments are the best forms of treatment.
- **Seborrhoeic dermatitis.** This condition is frequently confused with eczema, especially in younger children and babies. The common 'cradle-cap' seen in children under 1 year of age is an example of seborrhoeic dermatitis. In this condition the front of the child's hair is covered in a yellowish crust – even extending to the eyebrows at times – which, when gently removed, is seen to have a red, angry base. Other parts of the body can also be affected, such as the armpits, round chubby necks and the groin. Unlike eczema, this rash does not itch, and so secondary infection is not a problem. Treatment for cradle cap is to apply warm olive oil to the thick scales as a softening process before applying a specific cream to remove the surface skin. In other parts of the body a weak steroid cream is the better form of treatment. An antiseborrhoeic shampoo can also be of value. Seborrhoeic dermatitis is unusual in later childhood, but can return in later adult life.

SELF-HELP GROUP

National Eczema Society
163 Eversholt Street
London, NW1 1BU
Tel. 0171 388 4097.

ENURESIS

.

ALTERNATIVE NAME

Bed-wetting.

INCIDENCE

All young babies are wet at night as well as during the day. By 3 years of age, many children are dry by day and a few are also dry at night.

By 5 years of age most children have ceased wetting the bed except, perhaps, on a few occasions when sickening for a cold or some other infection, for example. There are, however, around 10% of children who are still enuretic at night on a regular basis. This figure falls to 1% or less by the time adolescence is reached.

Boys tend to take longer to achieve night-time bladder control than do girls.

CAUSATION

For convenience sake enuresis is divided into primary and secondary enuresis. Primary enuresis is said to occur when a child has never been dry at night apart from, possibly, a few odd occasions. Secondary enuresis is when a child who has previously been dry at night starts wetting again.

Primary enuresis may be due to a physical abnormality in the renal tract, or a neurological cause. It is important to exclude any such physical abnormality before commencing treatment for the enuresis. Developmental delay in this particular aspect of growing up may be the sole cause of the problem and is by far the commonest cause of primary enuresis.

Secondary enuresis is also common. There can frequently be found a precipitating cause for the onset again of bed-wetting after, perhaps, many months of dry beds. The arrival of a new baby, starting school, marital disharmony or the death of a grandparent are all examples of stressful events in the life of a child who only has precarious bladder control.

Social deprivation and low intelligence can also be possible factors in both forms of enuresis.

CHARACTERISTICS

This is obvious, and entails the child waking in the morning to find urine has been passed in the bed with no knowledge that this has happened. It is important that parents and child-carers understand that this is not a purposeful act on the part of the child just to be difficult. S/he is genuinely unaware that the bed is wet when waking initially in the morning. So punishment has absolutely no part to play in the treatment of enuresis.

Sometimes other factors noted in the child's **behaviour** are associated with the enuresis. For example, difficulties at school or temper tantrums can be signs that the child is under stress.

Daytime wetting is also found in some children with night-time enuresis. This can point to some abnormality in the renal tract or to a urinary infection. Both these conditions must be excluded before treatment of the enuresis is begun.

Enuresis also has a definite **familial pattern**. Parents of children with enuresis frequently admit to being late in achieving bladder control themselves. If this is the case, they will have a more sympathetic outlook on the problem than those parents who had no such bladder difficulties themselves when young.

INVESTIGATIONS

The **history** of the time of onset, duration and any treatment already tried must first of all be carefully ascertained.

Following this, all children with enuresis should have a **clinical examination** with special reference to the urinary tract and any possible neurological problems. Included in this examination, for example, must be palpation of the abdomen to be sure that the kidneys are not enlarged. If anything abnormal is discovered, an ultrasound examination is done. This will confirm the clinical findings.

The reflexes (for example, knee and ankle jerks) will give information on the normal, or otherwise, working of the nervous system, which is closely connected with bladder control.

A **sample of urine** must be sent to the laboratory to exclude any possible infection in the urinary tract that could have a bearing on the enuretic problem. A 'dip-stick' test of a sample of urine should also be done to exclude glycosuria (passing of excess sugar in the urine).

Enuresis is rarely – if ever – the sole sign of diabetes in a child but this, too, should be excluded as a possible cause for the bed-wetting.

MANAGEMENT

In all but around 1% of the 10% of children who are still wetting the bed at the age of 5 years, the problem will eventually resolve itself within a few years without any specific treatment. But much distress, to both mother and child, can occur along the way unless help is given. There are several paths that can be followed to speed up normal developmental progress of this particular aspect of growing up. Until around 5 years of age it is unwise to begin any systematic treatment. A relaxed attitude by parents, without censure for wet beds, will often result in a sudden succession of dry beds. Merely talking about the problem and learning how common it is can exert a magical effect on the whole family.

But if such simple measures have not succeeded, there are a number of ways in which help can be given.

'Star charts'

By the time the enuretic child has reached professional advice, this form of help – in one form or another – has often already been tried. Basically, the idea behind such charts is to encourage children to 'log' for themselves successful dry nights.

Enuresis clinics, which are run by some general practitioners and/or local authorities, will have available standard charts of various kinds. These all put emphasis on success rather than failure. In many cases this ritual, initiated by someone outside the immediate family, can be successful within a few weeks. If there is no, or little, success with this simple method after 3–4 months, other forms of treatment are indicated.

'Lifting' the child from sleep when parents go to bed and taking to the lavatory can be tried along with the star chart. Again, if no success is gained by this – or the child becomes distressed by being woken – it should be stopped.

Alarms

The alarm is probably one of the most well-known and advertised treatments for enuresis. This consists of a detector pad, powered by a battery, on which the child lies, separated by a sheet. If urine is passed through the sheet on to this pad the circuit is completed and the alarm sounds. There are a number of different types of alarms available. Some result in a loud buzzing noise when the circuit is completed (often waking the whole household!) while others only make a minimal sound from a device pinned to the child's nightclothes.

It is important that both mother and child should be shown together how to arrange and test the alarm. Failure to take time to do this can result in much disillusionment for both parent and child if the alarm fails to sound when urine has been passed in the night. It is important that follow-up, by someone skilled in the use of these alarms, is done on a regular basis. Minor adjustments, or repairs to the alarm, can make all the difference between success and failure.

In some parts of the country alarms can be borrowed from surgeries or local authority clinics. They can also be purchased in chemists or by mail order. If there has been no success with the alarm after 3 or 4 months of use, it is advisable to cease using this method for 6 months or so, and then to try again. Success rates with the alarm are good – around 80% – if used properly and with a positive attitude.

Other measures

Regular patterns of emptying the bladder during the day should be encouraged.

Emotional stress of any kind should be talked through with both parent and child. The causes of stress can be wide-ranging, from the trivial and easily corrected to the serious and potentially difficult to alter. If there are deep-seated problems, the help of a psychiatrist may be needed.

It may be helpful to suggest to the child a **goal** for becoming dry, such as, for example, a weekend camp or a visit to grandparents that includes an overnight stay. Such ruses, however, should be used with caution, as failure will cause further disillusionment.

There are two other forms of treatment that are sometimes suggested, both of which have limited success and are inadvisable.

- **Restriction of fluids during the day** only results in a thirsty child and a more irritable bladder due to concentrated urine. Obviously, a large drink just before bedtime is not a sensible idea, but the child should be allowed to drink as much as desired during the day.
- **Tricyclic antidepressants** have an initial success, but relapse almost invariably occurs once the medication is stopped.

THE FUTURE

Once dry beds have been achieved for a period of several weeks relapse rarely occurs – except perhaps temporarily at the onset of some infection.

The 1% of children who persist with enuresis into adolescence have difficult problems to overcome. All efforts must be made to ensure that no physical or emotional problems have been missed as a cause for the continuation of enuresis.

EPIGLOTTITIS

INCIDENCE

This is not exactly known. 'Epiglottitis' was only added, as a separate disease, to the OPCS tables between 1978 and 1980. Previously this condition was classified under the general heading of 'respiratory disorders'.

It is known, however, that 39 children died from epiglottitis in 1980. This sad figure has dropped over the years until in 1993 just two children died from the disease. Presumably, with specific recognition of the infection, specific treatment has been available, resulting in the gratifying fall in deaths.

Epiglottitis occurs in children between the ages of 2 and 7 years. The sexes are equally affected.

CAUSATION

Epiglottitis is an upper respiratory tract infection causing inflammation of the flap of tissue at the back of the throat known as the epiglottis. This important piece of tissue controls the passage of air into the lungs and the passage of food into the digestive system. So any swelling of the epiglottis can have far-reaching effects on both breathing and swallowing. In severe cases the passage of air into the lungs can be completely obstructed.

In the vast majority of cases the bacterium *Haemophilus influenzae* is the organism responsible for the infection. This organism can be isolated from throat swabs (but see below for the dangers of this procedure) or by blood culture from a child with an acute attack.

CHARACTERISTICS

Epiglottitis has an abrupt onset, and the child will become rapidly ill with:

- a **sore throat**;
- a **fever**;
- **difficulties in swallowing.**

This last symptom is quickly followed by **difficulties in breathing**. In contradistinction from an acute attack of croup, the child's breathing with epiglottis is **quiet and muffled**. (With croup the breathing is noisy and this is termed 'stridor'.) Because of the breathing problems the child's abdomen is indrawn with each breath, as can be also the neck above the collarbones. This is caused by the bringing into play of the accessory muscles of respiration – which are not normally used in breathing. It is only by this means that the child can get sufficient air into the lungs over the swollen and inflamed epiglottitis.

Within a few hours the child will become increasingly ill from the generalized toxic effects of the infection. Speaking is hoarse or impossible and **drooling** will result from the inability to swallow saliva. Breathing and pulse rates will rise and the child will become **exhausted** by the efforts needed to breathe. The child is also **restless** and **anxious**. Sitting up is the preferred position and often the **chin will be poked out** in an attempt to ease breathing.

Sudden **cessation of breathing** can occur as a result of complete blockage of the airway.

MANAGEMENT

Urgent **hospital admission** for paediatric intensive care is vital for a child with a severe attack of epiglottitis. If medical help is not quickly available, a 999 call is necessary. It is important that there is as little upset to the child as possible during the course of this procedure Even a minimal amount of distress can cause the onset of respiratory arrest. Any potentially unpleasant procedures, such as even the simple one of pushing down the tongue to see the throat, should be avoided.

In hospital, **intubation** – a tube passed down the throat to maintain an open airway – is the first priority. This will also allow the throat to be seen fully and so to confirm the diagnosis – this will be obvious when the cherry-red swelling at the base of the tongue is seen.

Intravenous antibiotics will need to be given as soon as possible.

The general condition of the child will also need to be closely **monitored** as septicaemia and/or pneumonia can occur as complications of this unpleasant, and potentially dangerous, disease.

COMPLICATIONS

Pneumonia can follow on from epiglottitis. If this happens there will be a deterioration of the child's general condition and a cough will become obvious. X-ray examination will show the extent of the problem.

Septicaemia – a generalized spread of the infection throughout the body via the blood-stream – is a further dangerous possibility, where again the child's general condition will worsen rapidly.

Meningitis can also occur. Headache, vomiting and stiffness of the child's neck will be the signs as well as, again, a worsening of the general condition.

These complications will all need specific and continuing hospital care.

THE FUTURE

Recovery from an uncomplicated attack of epiglottitis is quick and complete, there being no adverse after-effects.

Epilepsy

Alternative names

'The falling sickness'; fits; convulsions; seizures. (These three latter names are frequently used synonymously when discussing the manifestations due to epilepsy. This will apply in the following text.)

Incidence

Epilepsy can be defined as 'a recurrent sudden electrical discharge in the brain occurring in the absence of fever'. It is this abnormal discharge that produces the typical signs and symptoms of an epileptic seizure. The types of effect seen will depend on which part of the brain is affected. There can be generalized seizures affecting the whole body, and partial seizures affecting only certain parts or senses.

In school-age children, the incidence of epilepsy is between 4 and 9 in every 1000. (In preschool children, febrile convulsions – seen only in the under-fives – have a different incidence, aetiology and course. These convulsions are the direct effect of a sudden rise in temperature on the immature brain, and are grown out of by the fifth birthday. The incidence of febrile convulsions is around 3% of all preschool children.)

There are a number of conditions which, at first sight, can closely resemble epilepsy. For example breath-holding attacks and acute labyrinthitis can closely mimic an epileptic attack. These conditions must be carefully excluded before a diagnosis of epilepsy is made, with all the treatment and restrictions that such a diagnosis can imply.

Epilepsy is known in all countries of the world and affects both sexes.

History

Epilepsy has been described since biblical times, and, for many years, has unjustly stigmatized sufferers from this disorder. 'Devil-possessed' or 'mad' have frequently been descriptions applied to people suffering from epilepsy. Fortunately, today there is a better understanding of the cause and the course of this condition, together with successful drug treatments for the different types of epilepsy. But continuing further education of the public about these – often frightening to witness – episodes is still necessary.

Causation

Fits can be part of the symptomatology of complex **syndromes**, such as, for example, the Sturge–Weber syndrome and Batten's disease. (The figure of 140 genetic disorders associated with seizures has been quoted.)

Genetic inheritance appears to have a bearing on the occurrence of primary generalized – or idiopathic – epilepsy. It is thought that the risk of the children of epilepsy sufferers having the disorder is in the region of around 8%.

Developmental abnormalities in the structure of the brain can be the basis of the epilepsy. Some children who show generalized developmental delay can also have seizures as part of the general picture.

Chemical imbalance in the body can give rise to fits under certain conditions. For example, low calcium or magnesium levels can cause this problem, particularly in newborn babies, as can, under certain circumstances, low blood sugar. Fits due to these factors, however, cannot be classed as true epilepsy, as once the body physiology has been returned to normal the abnormal electrical activity will cease.

Seizures can also be a long-term complication following a **severe head injury.**

Infections, both those occurring prenatally, such as toxoplasmosis or infection with Cytomegalovirus, or those occurring later in childhood can be a cause of epilepsy. Such serious infections as meningitis, septicaemia or encephalitis can leave the child with recurrent seizures following recovery from the acute illness.

Tumours in the brain are a further cause of the onset of seizures in a child who has no previous history of epilepsy.

It can be seen that the list of possible causes of fits is almost as long as the types of fit themselves. So great care must be taken to attempt to determine a treatable cause for the fits before a diagnosis of idiopathic epilepsy is made – with all its future implications for treatment and lifestyle.

CHARACTERISTICS

Generalized seizures

These can be divided into 'grand mal', 'petit mal' and myoclonic seizures.

Grand mal epilepsy

This type of seizure occurs in about 80% of children who suffer from epilepsy. Before the fit, the child may behave in an unusual way or be especially irritable for some hours before the following sequence of events.

- There is a **sudden loss of consciousness** in which the child will fall to the ground and become rigid. At this time breathing will cease and the child will become blue through lack of oxygen. This is known as the **tonic phase** of a grand mal fit and lasts around 30 seconds.
- Following this there will be a phase – the **clonic phase** – in which the arms and legs will exhibit jerking movements. This phase is variable in length and can last several minutes. The movements will gradually cease and the child will slowly regain consciousness, having no memory of the seizure.

- Finally the child may feel the need to **sleep** for a variable length of time, or may be **confused** or **irritable** for a while.

Frothing at the mouth can occur at the height of the fit, and incontinence of urine may also occur. (Biting of the tongue is an extremely unusual occurrence in spite of the many lurid stories that abound!)

Petit mal

This type of epilepsy can be extremely difficult to diagnose. There are **short periods of altered consciousness** (10–15 seconds only) in which the child stops whatever s/he is doing and stares into space. Following this short period of 'absence', the activity or conversation will be picked up again as if there had been no interval. (A further – descriptive – name for petit mal is 'absences'.)

These absences can occur many times during the day. Often the only clue that they are occurring is a fall-off of the child's school performance. As a result of frequent absences, much can be missed over the course of a day's schooling. If this possibility is remembered, the child can be observed carefully and the attacks noted.

There are no involuntary movements or incontinence during these attacks of petit mal.

Myoclonic seizures

Myoclonic epilepsy most commonly occurs in children who have developmental delay, often due to underlying brain damage. The attacks are brief and may only consist of **jerking movements** of arms, body and/or legs. Occasionally only the head is involved in the jerky movement. The child may fall to the floor, but will recover quickly. (The Lennox–Gastaut syndrome – a specialized form of childhood epilepsy – commonly has myoclonic epilepsy as part of its symptomatology.)

Partial seizures

There are two main types of partial epileptic seizure. These arise as a result of abnormal electrical discharges in specific parts of the brain.

Rolandic epilepsy

Rolandic epilepsy (or **benign partial epilepsy of childhood**) occurs between the ages of 3 and 12 years. Symptoms occur most frequently at night, or during the period between sleeping and waking. This timing can make diagnosis difficult.

The child is conscious throughout the whole attack. S/he is often unable to speak, but will point to the side of the face, obviously trying to convey the unusual feelings that are occurring. During recovery, this area of the face may twitch. The whole episode is over within a couple of minutes.

Occasionally, unusual sensations of swelling or shrinking of an arm or one side of the face can be described afterwards by an articulate child.

The electroencephalogram (EEG) in this type of epilepsy shows a very typical diagnostic pattern. Fortunately, this benign type of epilepsy disappears completely around the age of 12–13 years, never to reappear. The abnormal EEG tracing gradually returns to normal.

Treatment is rarely necessary, but specific drugs will stop the attacks if they are occurring too frequently or the child is unduly distressed by them.

Temporal lobe epilepsy

Temporal lobe epilepsy is associated with a number of bizarre symptoms. The child may have specific hallucinations of a visual, auditory or olfactory nature. (A splendid old black and white film had as a main character someone who could smell fried onions as a prelude to his temporal lobe seizure!)

Alternatively, the sufferer may have sudden explosive attacks of rage or intense fear. Objective signs, such as flushing of the face, dilatation of the pupils of the eyes, or perspiration can also occur during an attack.

These occurrences are sometimes followed by a typical grand mal attack. Following the seizure the child feels confused and will need to sleep for an hour or more, although there is no definite memory of the attack.

These attacks are due to a number of possible factors, ranging from a previous severe infection, through a previous lack of oxygen causing damage to a specific part of the brain, to a cerebral tumour.

INVESTIGATIONS

A careful **history** of the attacks is the most important factor in the diagnosis of any form of epilepsy. The sequence of events as well as what actually happened – as described by a witness – will give clues as to whether the attack was epileptic or not.

Tests for chemical imbalances must be done on a sample of blood to exclude such conditions as diabetes or kidney failure, for example.

An **EEG** will show up any abnormalities in the brain waves. Many EEG patterns are quite specific for different forms of epilepsy.

CT scans are important follow-up investigations if it is thought that there is some physical abnormality in the brain causing the seizures.

Magnetic resonance imaging may, on occasions, be necessary to demonstrate a tiny lesion that could be missed on a CT scan.

All these investigations must, however, be interpreted in conjunction with a clear account of the actual seizure.

MANAGEMENT

Drugs

The decision to start drug treatment of epilepsy can be a difficult one. Rarely, if ever, are drugs needed for a single, or even two, seizures. But when attacks interfere with a child's everyday activities, drug treatment will be necessary – for example when there are so many 'absences' due to petit mal during a school day as to interfere with the child's ability to learn.

There is a wide range of drugs that can be used to control epilepsy. Each type of epilepsy has a drug, or group of drugs, that will best be able to control the seizures. In order to determine the drug best suited to each child's individual needs, it may be necessary to try various drugs, or two in combination. The most successful drug should then be prescribed on a long-term basis. Most children will need to take the drug of choice twice each day in order to control their fits adequately. It may be necessary to change the drug regimen as the child matures. Side-effects must also be noted, and regular measurements made of blood levels of the drug. Side-effects include giddiness, hyperactivity, headache, blurred vision and learning difficulties. These side-effects are quite specific to each drug.

Schooling

Children with epilepsy unrelated to any other pathological condition are quite able to attend an **ordinary school**. Figures quoted of the percentage of children with epilepsy normal in the intelligence range vary between 50% and 70%. The remainder of the children probably have a deficit in their intellectual ability due to other problems – which in themselves, of course, have a bearing on the aetiology of their seizures.

Teaching staff should be aware of their pupil's problems and be conversant with first aid treatment in case of a fit occurring during the school day. This latter event is, however, unlikely to occur if medication is carefully prescribed – and taken.

Some children will experience **learning difficulties** as a result of their epilepsy or associated disorders. Special schooling for these children will then be necessary.

Activities

Certain activities are dangerous for children with epilepsy.

- **Swimming** must always be in the presence of an adult who, ideally, should be in charge solely of the epileptic child.
- **Cycling** on the open road in fast-moving traffic should not be allowed.
- **Gymnastic activities** that necessitate climbing to a height up wall-bars or ropes should be forbidden. Other exercises in the gym are beneficial and should be encouraged.

Other measures

Family therapy, following the initial diagnosis, can be helpful if parents are particularly upset regarding the diagnosis. General practitioners, paediatricians, health visitors and teaching staff can all be involved in helping the family come to terms with the child's epilepsy. Full explanations of what is happening, the purpose of the treatment and how best to help the child live a happy, fulfilled life are all areas that will need to be explored.

Surgery plays a minor part in the management of epilepsy. This is restricted to helping uncontrollable epilepsy in some severely handicapped children.

The future

- **Driving**. A driving licence can be held by people with epilepsy provided that 2 years has elapsed without a daytime seizure – whether on medication or not.
- **Genetic counselling** before a pregnancy is undertaken may be necessary for some couples who have a strong family history of epilepsy.
- **Work**. Certain types of employment are inadvisable for people with epilepsy, e.g. work necessitating climbing to a height or working near to continuously moving machinery. Careers advice is helpful during the latter years at school.

Cessation of seizures

It has been estimated that by adulthood between 50% and 70% of children with epilepsy will have no further seizures. This, of course, is very much dependent upon the type and cause of the epilepsy.

SELF-HELP GROUPS

British Epilepsy Association
Gate Way Drive
Yeadon
Leeds, LS19 7XY
Tel. 0113 210 8800
Fax 0808 800 5050.

The National Society for Epilepsy
Chalfont St. Peter
Gerrards Cross, SL9 0RJ
Tel. 01494 601 300
Fax 01494 871 927.

Epilepsy Association of Scotland
48 Govan Road
Glasgow, G51 1JL
Tel. 0141 427 4911.

These associations provide support and information for teachers and families. Local conferences are arranged, as are holidays for children with severe epilepsy. There are information packs for schools as well as books, leaflets and videos on all aspects of epilepsy.

FIFTH DISEASE

ALTERNATIVE NAMES

'Slapped cheek syndrome'; erythema infectiosum.

INCIDENCE

This infection affects children between the ages of 2 and 10 years. Adults can also be affected, but this is unusual. For some unknown reason, girls are more frequently affected than boys.

Outbreaks of this condition can occur at any time of the year but are most common during the winter and the spring. This is in line with the higher incidence of many infections due to the closer proximity of children to one another during the colder months of the year.

CAUSATION

Fifth disease is caused by a virus of the Parvovirus group. The infection is spread from child to child by droplet infection. The virus is also thought to be contracted from infected blood products when, for example, a child has a blood transfusion for some reason. The incubation period is variable, anything from 5–20 days after exposure being quoted.

CHARACTERISTICS

Frequently the first sign of the 'slapped cheek syndrome' is the typical **rash** (similar in type to that seen in rubella) that appears on the child's cheeks. As the name implies, it appears as if the child has received a blow to the face. (Fifth disease must always be remembered as a possibility when there has been a previous high index of suspicion of child abuse.)

In contrast to the bright red rash on the cheeks, the area around the child's mouth is seen to be **pale**. (A similar phenomenon is seen in scarlet fever. This latter infection is, however, a far more serious and severe disease, and the two infections are distinguished by the more generalized and serious constitutional upset seen in scarlet fever.) In 2 or 3 days the rash extends to the chest and limbs. This lasts for a week or two and then gradually fades, but can be seen to return for a further couple of weeks on the child having a hot bath. This rash can be mildly irritating.

There may also be a **fever** associated with the illness, this usually being in evidence before the rash appears. This, as with all feverish illness, is associated with **headache** and a general feeling of **malaise** and **aching limbs.**

INVESTIGATIONS

Blood tests: The diagnosis can be confirmed by a specialized laboratory test on a sample of blood. This is rarely performed in an uncomplicated case of fifth disease, but may be necessary if any of the rare complications occur.

MANAGEMENT

As with most viral infections, there is no specific treatment, antibiotics being of no value in infections of viral origin.

Analgesics, for control of fever, if present to any degree, and to relieve headaches and aching limbs, should be given if necessary. Dosage must, of course, be appropriate to the age of the child. (Aspirin must not be given to children under the age of 12 years because of the link between this analgesic and Reye's syndrome.)

It is not necessary to keep a child with fifth disease away from **school** unless s/he is feeling too unwell due to fever and other symptoms of infection. As infection is passed on from child to child before the rash appears, staying away from school will not help reduce the spread of the infection. Once the rash has appeared, the child is no longer infectious.

COMPLICATIONS

A mild **arthritis** can occur with the slapped cheek syndrome, usually beginning a few days before the appearance of the rash. Although this complication more commonly occurs in adults with the infection, children can also suffer. The pain associated with the arthritis tends to come and go in a fleeting fashion, and can last many weeks. The smaller joints are usually affected – fingers, wrists and ankles. Analgesics may be necessary to control this pain.

There are two **special groups of children** who have complications due to fifth disease. One of these comprises those who have **thalassaemia** or **sickle cell anaemia**. Here the infection may precipitate a 'crisis' in which levels of haemoglobin fall dangerously low. Blood transfusion may be necessary for these children until the effects of the virus have worn off. The other group of children who can suffer from complications comprises those children with a pre-existing malignancy, particularly **acute leukaemia**. Specialized treatment is necessary under these conditions.

PREVENTION

There is no immunization available against the slapped cheek syndrome.

THE FUTURE

There is no long-term disability following an attack of fifth disease. The arthritis that sometimes occurs is only temporary and does not recur in later life. If the disease is contracted during pregnancy, miscarriage can occur, but this is not invariably so.

GASTROENTERITIS

INCIDENCE

Gastroenteritis is one of the commonest of childhood infections. This is so throughout the world. While the incidence of this illness has fallen steadily in the West, in many developing countries gastroenteritis is still one of the major killer diseases in children. The dramatic fall in fatalities in the West due to this infection has largely been brought about by improved hygiene and the energetic treatment of dehydration in children with an acute attack of gastroenteritis.

Outbreaks of gastroenteritis still occur, however, in nurseries and schools, with isolated incidents in homes throughout the country – 50% of the cases occurring in children below the age of 5 years. This is especially so in the winter months, when close contact among children is more usual than in the summer months.

HISTORY

Diarrhoeal diseases have always been a problem where large numbers of people congregate together. Cholera, dysentery and typhoid were common gastrointestinal disorders during the last century. Since that time public health measures regarding purity of drinking water and disposal of sewage have transformed the picture in developed countries.

CAUSATION

Gastroenteritis can be caused by bacteria or viruses. It is thought that around 50% of all gastroenteritis attacks are caused by the Rotavirus. These tiny viruses were first detected in Australia. They can be visualized under the electron microscope.

The infection is probably passed from child to child by imperfect hand-washing after visiting the lavatory, for example. Perhaps the infection can also be passed on by droplet infection from the respiratory tract – many children with a diarrhoeal disease have also had a cold a few days previously. Children up to the age of 6 years are particularly prone to gastroenteritis due to these viruses. After this age, the majority of children have built up an immunity to the virus and so do not suffer from symptoms of the infection.

The Norwalk virus is one of the more publicized viruses causing gastroenteritis in recent years. But there are a number of other viruses which also cause similar unpleasant symptoms.

There are also several bacteria causing gastroenteritis. The commonest of these are the *Escherichia coli* (*E. coli*), *Salmonella* and *Shigella* bacteria. The fall of gastroenteritis cases in the West is largely due to better control of these bacteria. Outbreaks of *Salmonella* still occur, and are usually due to contaminated food. Contact tracing of these outbreaks is energetically pursued and appropriate steps are taken to improve hygiene to avoid further problems.

CHARACTERISTICS

Whatever the causative organism, the clinical signs and symptoms of an acute attack of gastroenteritis are similar.

The early stages of the infection can well be non-specific. The baby or young child will be **irritable, cry** and cease to play happily. Food will be refused, and an excessive thirst may be noticed.

Within a few hours, **vomiting** will occur, especially in younger children. This will usually precede the **diarrhoea**, which soon follows. (These symptoms can also, of course, occur in other conditions, which need surgery – e.g. appendicitis and intussusception.) **Fever** is variable – sometimes only a mild fever is present, while at other times the temperature is high. This latter occurs more frequently with an infection by the Rotavirus group.

INVESTIGATIONS

Usually – and fortunately – attacks of gastroenteritis in children are short-lived and mild. In these cases, no investigation into the causative organism is necessary. But if an outbreak in a nursery or a school, for example, occurs, samples of the stools of sufferers and their families should be sent to the laboratory for identification of the infecting organism.

MANAGEMENT

Toddlers and older children

In **mild cases** where vomiting and frequent diarrhoea is not a serious problem, **fluids only** should be given for 24 hours. In the young child this is usually no problem, as food is the last thing s/he will wish to see or take! Plain water, or water with the addition of a teaspoon of glucose to a glass, whenever thirst is complained of is all that is necessary for 24 hours. Following this, provided that vomiting has ceased and the diarrhoea has improved, solid food can be reintroduced gradually over the next few days.

In more severe cases, **replacement of lost fluid** by one of the commercial replacement fluids (obtainable from chemists) will be necessary. Again, no solid food should be given.

Medical advice should always be sought if the diarrhoea and vomiting is severe and/or persists for longer than a few hours. This is especially important in young children. Large amounts of fluid can be lost by severe diarrhoea and vomiting and small children cannot easily replace this loss.

Hospital admission may be necessary for the small child with a severe attack of gastroenteritis, because of this fluid loss. Under these circumstances, not only is the loss of fluid itself potentially dangerous but the blood chemistry can be seriously disarranged. Skilled medical and nursing care are required.

Babies under 1 year

Similar treatment is necessary for small babies as for older children. But it must be remembered that tiny babies become dehydrated very quickly and can become dangerously ill in a very short time. So medical advice must be obtained quickly for these little ones.

Kaolin, or any of the other antidiarrhoeal agents, is of no value in childhood gastroenteritis.

Antibiotics are also of no value in gastroenteritis due to a virus, but should be used in proven cases of *Salmonella* infection.

COMPLICATIONS

Dehydration, as described above, is the most immediate and serious complication. Treatment is as described, but with more emphasis on early medical help the younger the child.

Sugar intolerance is a common complication following an attack of gastroenteritis. The younger the child, the more frequently this occurs. Symptoms appear as soon as milk is reintroduced into the diet following the initial treatment. Diarrhoea will again become a problem, with frequent, frothy, watery stools that in turn often give rise to an unpleasant nappy-rash. (It is the sugar – lactose – in the milk that causes the problem.) The basic cause of this temporary intolerance is the damage done to the lining of the intestine by the bacteria or virus causing the gastroenteritis.

Treatment is to give a lactose-free milk for a few weeks to give the intestine time to recover. After about 4–6 weeks ordinary milk should be gradually reintroduced into the diet, and usually there is no return of the diarrhoea. If there is, the process should be repeated until ordinary milk is tolerated again.

PREVENTION

It would be good to think that all attacks of gastroenteritis in children – and adults – could be prevented. Unfortunately it is difficult to imagine this scenario, although work is proceeding towards a vaccine against the Rotavirus.

Good hygiene in the preparation of food and instillation of regular hand-washing after visiting the lavatory and before meals is important in controlling the spread of infection.

Medical advice should be obtained sooner, rather than later, especially in the case of young babies, in order to prevent complications.

GLANDULAR FEVER

ALTERNATIVE NAMES

Infectious mononucleosis; 'kissing disease'.

INCIDENCE

Glandular fever is usually a disease affecting older children and young adolescents. But younger children are by no means immune to the condition, although children under the age of 3 years rarely suffer from the disease.

Overcrowding and poor hygiene are factors in the spread of the infection, which is passed on by close physical contact. The virus is harboured in the throat and salivary glands – often for many months after recovery from the original infection. (This is the reason for the popular name – 'kissing disease' – of glandular fever, and is the most likely form of spread during the adolescent years.) Epidemics can also occur in schools and residential homes.

There is no particular time of the year when glandular fever is more common, cases occurring throughout the seasons.

The infection is worldwide, and is no respecter of the sexes.

HISTORY

The incidence of glandular fever appears to have changed since the earlier days of the 20th century. At this time, younger children were the most frequent sufferers, and epidemics among this age group were described. These are no longer seen to occur.

CAUSATION

Glandular fever is caused by a virus of the herpes group – the Epstein–Barr virus. The incubation period is thought to be between 5 and 10 days. But because the virus remains in the throat and salivary glands, infection in a second person can occur up to 12 weeks after the initial attack.

CHARACTERISTICS

Glandular fever can be notoriously difficult to diagnose clinically. This is partly because there are a number of different ways in which the infection can manifest itself. Also, signs and symptoms at times are very similar to other infective conditions, such as tonsillitis or influenza.

Characteristically, however, glandular fever begins with **tiredness** and a general feeling of **malaise** with **headache, muscular pains, sore throat and fever** – all very general signs of any infectious illness. In glandular fever, however, many of the **glands in the neck** become swollen. Swelling of the **glands in the armpit and groin** soon follow.

Occasionally in children there is a transient **rash** at the onset of the disease. (If ampicillin, an antibiotic commonly used to control infections, is given to a child who has glandular fever, a severe rash can be the result.)

The **tonsils** are seen to be red and swollen (a very similar picture to that seen in an attack of tonsillitis). Swallowing can be difficult for the youngster in severe cases.

On close examination of the mouth, the **palate** is seen to have tiny haemorrhages in the early stages of the infection. This sign is specific to glandular fever, and can help to make the diagnosis clear if seen early enough in the infection.

The **spleen** is enlarged and often tender to touch. Also, the **liver** is often enlarged, and **jaundice** may be a feature.

INVESTIGATIONS

Blood tests show a specific feature with an excess in the number of a particular type of white cell. A specific test on the blood – the Paul–Bunnell reaction – confirms the diagnosis of glandular fever, but is only positive in 60% of cases. There is a similar rapid slide test – the 'Monospot' test – which can be performed quickly in the surgery without the need to wait for laboratory results. Both these tests can be negative in the early stages of the disease – yet a further complication – but will be positive if repeated a week later.

Other **specific laboratory tests** done on a blood sample will show changes that will help with the diagnosis.

MANAGEMENT

There is no specific treatment for an attack of glandular fever. Acyclovir – a useful drug against some viral infections under certain conditions – is of no value against infection with the Epstein–Barr virus.

Rest (not necessarily in bed), with **adequate fluids** and a **light diet**, together with analgesics to relieve the pain of the sore throat and headache and plenty of sympathy is all that can be done.

A **throat swab** should be taken if the tonsillar involvement is severe and the glands in the neck are tender as well as swollen. At times, a secondary infection with *Streptococcus* bacteria can add to the patient's miseries. Under these circumstances, treatment with penicillin is indicated.

Most children will completely recover from an attack of glandular fever within 3 weeks. But occasionally the feelings of malaise, mild fever and lack of appetite can drag on for weeks or months. Under these conditions it is wise to for a chest X-ray to be taken to exclude any further infection in the lungs.

Difficulties can arise in older children if they succumb to an attack of glandular fever at **examination times**. There is no doubt that the child will not be able to give of his/her best if s/he has only recently recovered from glandular fever. Most educational authorities recognize this and make the appropriate allowances.

COMPLICATIONS

Secondary bacterial infection can occur in throat or chest, as mentioned above, and must be treated with the appropriate antibiotic.

Liver involvement, giving rise to jaundice, rarely occurs in children. If, however, it does, recovery will be complete and rapid.

Occasionally there can be a **relapse**, with symptoms similar to the original attack after a few weeks. Again, this will resolve spontaneously with a few days rest.

PREVENTION

Sensible precautions, such as good hygiene, avoidance of overcrowding and minimal close contact with the sufferer is all that can be done by way of preventative measures.

THE FUTURE

There are no long-term after-effects from glandular fever.

HAND, FOOT AND MOUTH SYNDROME

INCIDENCE

Small outbreaks of this graphically named infection can occur among babies and older children. The summer months are the most likely time for the condition to occur. Adults can suffer from the disease as well as children.

HISTORY

Hand, foot and mouth disease was first recognized as a clinical entity in Toronto in 1957. An outbreak of the infection occurred with quite specific features, and was named according to the characteristics noted. (The name bears an unfortunate resemblance to the foot and mouth disease found in cattle – but has absolutely nothing to do with this!)

CAUSATION

Hand, foot and mouth disease is caused by a virus of the Coxsackie group. The virus can be isolated from the skin lesions and also from the stools of sufferers.

The incubation period for this infection is unknown.

CHARACTERISTICS

There may be a mild constitutional upset before the typical rash appears. The child may have a **mild fever**, and complain of a **headache** and a general feeling of **malaise**.

Babies may be reluctant to take their feeds, and older children be unwilling to eat as the rash starts to make its appearance.

The **rash** is very specific and consists of small, greyish-white, blistery spots with a surrounding red halo. These are found on the tongue, making this mobile organ sore. The palms of the hands and the sides of the soles of the feet are also affected. Occasionally this rash may become more widespread, and can often be seen to cover the buttocks as well. (If the rash does occur on the buttocks, confusion can arise between this condition and Henoch–Schönlein purpura – see below.)

The rash lasts between 3 and 5 days and then fades rapidly. Other symptoms, if present, then also improve rapidly and the child is restored to full health.

Management

General sympathetic care is all that is required for an attack of hand, foot and mouth disease. **Fluids only** for a day or two may be required if the child's mouth is sore following the appearance of the rash. Otherwise, **bland foods** will be better tolerated than spicy, highly flavoured ones until the tongue has returned to normal.

Analgesics to reduce fever and relieve headache should be given if necessary. Paracetamol compounds only should be given to children, as aspirin runs the risk, in under-12-year-olds, of Reye's syndrome.

School-age children should **remain away from school** while the rash is present on their hands. As the incubation period of this infection is unknown, the time when it can be passed on is uncertain, but, as with most viral infections, the most infectious period is probably the time just before the rash appears.

Complications

The only complication that has been reported to occur with this infection is for the rash to **extend all over the body**. This is rare, but must be remembered when a child is seen with a rash that covers the whole of the body. The diagnosis can be made by the very obvious greyish rash that covers the palms of the hands and soles of the feet.

The future

There are no long-term effects in later life from hand, foot and mouth disease.

HAY-FEVER

ALTERNATIVE NAME

Seasonal allergic rhinitis.

INCIDENCE

It is thought that between 10% and 20% of the population suffer from hay-fever. The time of the year at which the symptoms appear is dependent upon which particular tree or flower produces the allergy in each individual person.

Springtime – March to May – when many plants come into bloom shows the highest incidence of hay-fever. Late flowering plants such as carnations, dahlias and chrysanthemums, as well as the common stinging nettle, can all produce symptoms later in the year, from July to September. Moulds and mildews, usually at their height during warm, damp weather, can also affect some people. So, while hay-fever (as its name implies) is at its height during the spring, certain sufferers are not immune for the rest of the year.

Hay-fever affects both sexes equally and even young children can be affected, although most children begin to suffer first of all during the early school years.

Afro-Caribbean children living in the UK appear to have a higher incidence of hay-fever than average. It has also been reported that children of non-manual workers are more prone to hay-fever.

CAUSATION

Hay-fever is the third member of the allergy trio: asthma, eczema and hay-fever. The cause is an allergic reaction to the pollens of many different types of tree, grass and flowers of all kinds. The amount of pollen produced by just one flower is incredible – one flower of sorrel being reported as producing 180 000 grains of pollen. In a high wind these grains can be carried for more than 10 miles! Difficult indeed to take avoiding action from the effects of these minute grains of pollen.

Susceptibility to these allergens is often inherited. Other members of the family may not themselves be hay-fever sufferers, but may have asthma or eczema.

Symptoms, of course, are at their worst when the pollen count is high.

CHARACTERISTICS

- Profuse clear, watery **discharge from the nose**, often associated with sneezing.

- **Red, runny, itchy eyes.** This symptom is sometimes known by the alternative name of 'allergic conjunctivitis' and can occur without the other symptoms of hay-fever. The causative factors are similar.
- **Wheezing and breathlessness** can also occur with hay-fever as well as asthma. The differential diagnosis between these two conditions can at times be blurred.
- **Itching of the soft palate** (and also at times the **ears**, due to a common nerve supply between these two structures).

Diagnosis is based on the occurrence of these symptoms at times of the year that are specific to each sufferer.

MANAGEMENT

It is virtually impossible to avoid contact with pollen altogether. Even if this were possible, it would be hard to keep children indoors during the warm summer months. There are a number of drug treatments available that will subdue most of the symptoms of hay-fever.

- **Eye-drops of sodium cromoglycate** – the same drug that is used as a prophylactic measure in asthma – are very successful in keeping the eye symptoms under control. The drops will need to be instilled on a regular basis four times a day. This regimen needs to be strictly adhered to throughout the hay-fever season.
- **Antihistamines** (there are those available that do not cause drowsiness) are helpful for mild cases, and again should be used throughout the season.
- **Steroids used in an inhaler** are necessary for more severe cases.
- **Steroids given in tablet form** by mouth can be used in the short term for children with disabling symptoms of hay-fever. These drugs (which are not advised for long-term use) are useful to tide a teenager with severe hay-fever over a difficult examination period.

THE FUTURE

Some sufferers find that their hay-fever improves as the years go by, but most children suffering from hay-fever will continue to do so throughout their lives. It is fortunate that there are drugs available to control the symptoms.

Headache

Incidence

Headaches are a surprisingly common symptom in children. By the age of 10 years it is thought that around 10% of all children have headaches of a recurring nature. A further piece of research in children under the age of 5 years found that 19% had complained of a headache. (Young children often do not have the verbal skills to describe their pain, but comments such as 'My head is sore' or 'My head bangs' are common, while other children show their distress by holding their heads or burying them in a pillow.)

Headaches are often part and parcel of other illnesses, the associated symptoms of which override the pain of the headache. For example the fever and rash of an infectious childhood illness, such as chickenpox, will take precedence over the headache, although this is undoubtedly present.

Causation

Headaches can be divided into three main causative groups:

- **vascular** (related to the blood system) **headaches** – migraine is the classical example of this type of headache;
- **'tension' headaches**;
- **headaches associated with other illnesses**. This last group can be further subdivided into those headaches that have an infection as their prime cause and those due to other problems, such as brain tumours or previous head injury.

There is a further small subgroup of conditions that can give rise to pain which children can describe as a 'headache'. This includes the facial pain of sinusitis and visual difficulties, such as unrecognized short-sightedness.

Headaches in children are a worrying symptom for parents. At the back of everyone's mind is the thought of serious conditions, such as a brain tumour or meningitis. While these are comparatively rare reasons for a headache, medical advice should be sought sooner rather than later. This is particularly important if the headache is severe and/or it lasts longer than 3–4 hours or is associated with other symptoms, such as vomiting and/or fever.

Characteristics

Vascular headaches are those that cause migraine. This is fully described under Migraine, below.

Tension headaches have different characteristics from those of migraine. They tend to be more continuous, not occurring in definite episodes as does migraine. The headache is usually **present every day** and often **persists throughout the day** at varying levels of pain or discomfort.

Headaches of this type are not usually as severe as the pain of a full-blown attack of migraine. Children often describe this type of headache as a tight **band around the head**. Also, pain in the muscles at the **back of the neck** can be a feature. Unlike migraine, there is no visual disturbance or vomiting.

With this type of headache it is worth making enquiries into the child's activities and behaviour at nursery or school. A specific **learning difficulty** or other worrying aspect of school life, such as **bullying**, can be the basic cause of this type of headache.

Children, too, as well as adults, can suffer from **depression** – perhaps more frequently than is realized. Marital discord, step-family difficulties, and bereavement by the death of a close family member can all be causes of understandable depression, which can be manifested as a tension headache. Other more subtle reasons, such as fear of the dark or a worrying television programme, for example, must be remembered when attempting to sort out the cause of a tension headache.

Headaches associated with other illnesses can again be subdivided into three distinct categories.

- Those infectious illnesses – influenza, a common cold, chickenpox, for example – that involve a **fever** are all associated to headache of some degree. This symptom may be one of the child's least concerns when all limbs ache, everywhere is hot and sticky and, to add to the miseries, an itchy rash appears! Nevertheless, if questioned specifically, the presence of a headache will be agreed.
- More seriously, there are those headaches that are caused by a **brain tumour**. Under these circumstances the headache is usually **worse in the mornings** when the child wakes. **Sleep** may also have been disturbed by the pain of the headache – in fact, the mere act of lying down can at times worsen the pain. Headaches due to this cause tend to be **continuous**, with exacerbation of the severity of the pain under the conditions mentioned. There may also be other signs of the underlying problem, e.g. some specific **muscle weakness** or **double vision**, depending on the actual position of the tumour. **Convulsions** can also occur, as can also subtle changes in **personality** or **behaviour**.
- Headaches can also occur some time after a **head injury**. Here bleeding has occurred beneath one particular layer of the membranes covering the brain. The subsequent blood clot – known as a **subdural haematoma** – will press on the surrounding tissue, giving rise to a headache. Dangerous further **bleeding** can occur at a later date under these circumstances.

If any of these conditions is suspected, further investigations – a **scan** and maybe **magnetic resonance imaging** – will need to be done urgently. Following the results of these tests, appropriate treatment – surgical or chemical – will need to be instituted.

MANAGEMENT

Basically, the treatment of a headache must be that of the underlying cause, with the addition of a drug such as **paracetamol** – in appropriate dosage for the child's age – to subdue the pain until specific treatment can be given.

Tension headaches need careful and sympathetic investigation into the possible cause of **stress**. As previously mentioned, enquiries into any problems – whether of learning or social contact – arising during a school day need to be made. Children are often reluctant to tell parents of difficulties that they may be having at school – if indeed they are even aware of what exactly is the matter. At times, the help of an **educational psychologist** will need to be enlisted if learning difficulties are a possibility.

It is counter-productive to keep a child with a tension-type headache away from **school**. Lessons will be missed and so cause extra stress when these have to be made up. Also of importance is to be sure that both child and parents know that tension headaches are not serious and not an indication of any later sinister disease.

Headaches due to intercurrent illness, such as a cold or flu, will improve once the disease has run its course. Paracetamol will help reduce the pain of the associated headache as well as lowering temperature and improving the pain of aching limbs.

Headaches due to brain tumours or subdural haematoma need special investigations and treatments appropriate to each individual cause.

To summarize, headaches in children need **further investigation** if:

- the headache is **worse in the mornings** when awakening from sleep;
- the headache is worse when the child **coughs**;
- the headache **wakes** the child or **prevents sleep**;
- there is **weakness, numbness** or **tingling** in any part of the body in association with the headache;
- persistent **vomiting** occurs with the headache;
- there is any **change in the child's personality or behaviour.**

Henoch–Schönlein purpura

Alternative name

Anaphylactoid purpura.

Incidence

There are no available figures for this condition, but it is not an especially common disorder. Nevertheless when it does occur the signs and symptoms are sufficiently severe to cause alarm and – at times – difficulties in diagnosis.

Henoch–Schönlein purpura can run a protracted course, with associated implications for both care and education. Fortunately, full recovery – in a time scale ranging from 6 weeks to 1 year – is the usual outcome of this disease.

The condition is commonest among preschool children, even as young as 1 year, but all age groups can be affected.

Boys are more frequently affected than girls.

History

The double barrelled name of this disease arose due to the involvement of two doctors – Henoch and Schönlein – in the description of the condition. Henoch described the relationship of the specific rash with the gastrointestinal symptoms, while Schönlein placed emphasis on the relationship of the rash with the arthritic manifestations. It was later realized that both descriptions related to the one disease.

Causation

The basic cause of Henoch–Schönlein purpura is unknown, but it probably results from an immune system problem.

The pathology is one of inflammation around the capillaries and small arteries (a vasculitis) in many – and varied – parts of the body, including the skin, the gastrointestinal tract and the kidneys.

There have been suggestions that the onset of the condition may be preceded by an upper respiratory tract infection, but this is not always the case.

Characteristics

The typical **rash** is usually the first sign of the disease. This rash consists of small 'bruise-like' ('purpuric') spots around a blistery centre. This rash, unlike a number of other rashes, does not disappear when pressed with a finger. It is the result of the inflammatory process around the blood vessels.

The distribution of the rash is quite distinctive, being mainly confined to the backs of the legs and the buttocks. In some children the rash may be minimal and confined to only a few spots. But if they are seen in a child who is complaining of the other typical symptoms, the diagnosis is made clear.

The rash is painless and does not itch. As fading takes place over the succeeding days, the typical yellow discoloration seen on a fading bruise is seen.

Gastrointestinal tract

Symptoms in this body system are often the most unpleasant ones in Henoch–Schönlein purpura. Because of the lesions – similar to the ones seen on the skin – in the intestine, bleeding occurs. This gives rise to **colicky abdominal pain,** which can either be persistent or come and go intermittently. Acute abdominal pain in children is notoriously difficult to diagnose, as there are a multitude of possible causes. It is the relationship with the skin rash that provides the clue to the diagnosis of Henoch–Schönlein purpura. **Vomiting** can also occur in association with the abdominal pain.

Blood in the motions is a common feature, although this may not be obvious to the naked eye. Laboratory testing will confirm that bleeding has occurred into the intestine.

Children with this kind of continuing abdominal pain will often become unduly **depressed** – understandably so. There is nothing quite so lowering as continuing tummy pain.

Joints

Some joints of the body can be affected. The child will complain of **pain and tenderness,** particularly on movement. This pain, as with the abdominal pain, can be intermittent. This is again due to the inflammation of the small blood vessels around the affected joints.

Renal tract

The kidneys can also be specifically involved in Henoch–Schönlein purpura. This is an especially worrying aspect of this otherwise benign disease. Long-term effects can result from the involvement of the renal tract. Again, as in the gastrointestinal tract, there can be bleeding from the small blood vessels in the renal tract. This bleeding again may not be visible in the child's urine to the naked eye, but can be demonstrated by laboratory testing. Associated with this is the passage of microscopic amounts of protein in the urine, again demonstrable in the laboratory.

The timing of the renal tract involvement can be unusual, occasionally arising as late as 3 months after the appearance of the rash. So it is important that a check should be kept on the child's urine at intervals for several months after an attack of Henoch–Schönlein purpura. (In a few – very rare – cases, the kidney involvement is a major feature of the disease, and runs a rapidly downhill course leading to fatal renal failure.)

Henoch–Schönlein purpura is a condition that can resolve completely within 6 weeks, leaving the child in complete health. There can also be remissions back into abdominal and joint pain for as long as 1 year with protein also continuing to be excreted in the urine, showing that the kidneys are still being affected by the disease. But in the vast majority of cases recovery is eventually complete, with no long-lasting ill effects.

INVESTIGATIONS

Blood tests show few specific changes in an attack of Henoch–Schönlein purpura.

Urine testing, as mentioned, shows varying amounts of protein and/or blood according to the degree to which the kidneys are involved in the condition.

MANAGEMENT

While there are no specific drugs that will produce a dramatic cure, careful management of the – sometimes very distressing – symptoms of the disease is important.

Bed rest during the period when the rash is at its height is advised. It has been found that the rash tends to worsen if the child is allowed to run around. Also, if there is obvious bleeding from the renal tract, bed rest is advisable.

Analgesics to control the pain from tender joints will give much relief. The abdominal pain can also be controlled by analgesics. In mild cases paracetamol will suffice, but children with severe abdominal pain will need stronger drugs to control this distressing symptom. Occasionally, steroids will be needed to give relief.

Emotional support for both parents and child during the possibly long-drawn-out process of this disease is important. Full explanations of the possible cause and probable sequence of events should be given, so that parents can cope with each new manifestation if, or when, it arises The child's possible depression also needs to be discussed, and plans made to mitigate this as far as possible.

Schooling can be resumed when the rash has disappeared and pain is absent from joints. Because of the possible relapsing course of this disease, teachers should be kept advised of problems as they arise. Work may need to be sent home if the child is not up to coping with the rough and tumble of the school day. School staff should also be reassured that the condition is not infectious.

Regular **review of kidney function**, together with blood pressure meaurements, should be done until all signs of protein in the urine are absent.

COMPLICATIONS

The important complication of continuing renal involvement must always be borne in mind. **Hypertension** (high blood pressure) can result from severe involvement of the kidneys. If this occurs, it should be treated to avoid further problems in later life.

The **nephrotic syndrome**, in which there is continuing, and excessive, amounts of protein excreted in the urine, together with marked swelling of various of parts of the body, can also – but rarely – result from an attack of Henoch–Schönlein purpura.

THE FUTURE

Henoch–Schönlein purpura is rarely fatal. But if renal involvement has been severe, high blood pressure may be a problem in later life.

Impetigo

Incidence

Impetigo is a well-known skin disease worldwide. Latterly – in the past decade – there has been an increase in the type of impetigo caused by a specific bacterium, *staphylococcus*, with a decrease in impetigo caused by other bacteria.

Children are especially prone to this skin infection.

Causation

Impetigo can be caused by either *Staphylococcus* or *Streptococcus* bacteria. As mentioned above, there has been a worldwide increase lately in impetigo caused by *staphylococci*. Streptococcal impetigo is rarely seen nowadays. This has a bearing on the type of treatment necessary to cure the infection.

Impetigo often arises following other skin diseases such as eczema, scabies or even a minor insect bite. Scratching induced by these other skin conditions allows the bacteria to enter the abraded surface of the skin.

Characteristics

Impetigo is an infection of the skin. Initially a small, blistery spot appears. The area around the mouth and nose is most frequently affected, although theoretically any part of the body can be affected. The skin in these former areas is more liable to infection because of the general soreness and irritation, with subsequent rubbing, caused by the common cold.

The initial sore spot increases with sometimes alarming rapidity, both in size and in the number of lesions.

Within a few hours, the surface of the skin breaks down, leaving a raw, moist surface that quickly becomes crusted over. In a particular subtype of impetigo, much serum is exuded from the broken-down rash. This forms a thick, yellow crust over an underlying reddened, sore area.

Impetigo is a **highly contagious** condition. In spite of the alarming sight of the rash of impetigo, this infection is not painful or itchy, and there is rarely any associated generalized systemic upset.

As the rash clears following treatment, superficial skin cells can sometimes be shed, leaving a raw area for a short time. This is known as the 'scalded skin syndrome' or Lyell's disease. The rash of impetigo fortunately leaves no permanent scarring.

INVESTIGATIONS

Ideally, a swab should be taken from the weeping lesion of impetigo and sent to the laboratory so that the invading organism can be identified. From this information the most suitable antibiotic can then be prescribed. This is especially important if a number of children – in a class for example – are involved, or if the treatment given is not proving to be successful.

MANAGEMENT

As impetigo is caused by bacteria, **antibiotics** will soon clear the unpleasant rash. While sensitivities to the particular organism are being awaited (or if no swab has been able to be taken) erythromycin, given by mouth, is one of the most useful antibiotics. In early stages, or where only a small area of skin is involved, an antibiotic cream may be sufficient to produce a cure.

School, and contact with other children, **should be avoided** until the lesions have completely cleared. Because of its highly infectious nature, impetigo can spread like wildfire around a class of schoolchildren or a nursery. This is particularly so among the younger age groups, partly because of their incomplete knowledge of hygiene at this age!

COMPLICATIONS

On the rare occasions that the group A *Streptococcus* bacterium is the cause of the impetigo, watch should be kept, for around 2 months after the infection, for possible **kidney involvement**. Signs of this will be:

- blood in the urine;
- swelling of tissues, particularly around the face;
- a decrease in the amount of urine passed.

This is a serious condition, and one which must receive urgent treatment. It must be stressed, however, that this is extremely rare – especially as impetigo due to streptococcal bacteria is unusual these days.

Impetigo may complicate a pre-existing eczema.

THE FUTURE

There are no long-term after-effects of an uncomplicated attack of impetigo. The condition can recur, as immunity to the bacteria is not gained by the one attack.

INTUSSUSCEPTION

INCIDENCE

Intussusception is essentially a condition seen in infancy, 3–9 months being the most usual time for this to occur. It can occur in older children, but the reasons for this happening are usually different from those occurring in infancy.

Some authorities consider that the incidence is markedly higher in boys than in girls – the ratio being as much as 5:1. Other professionals consider the incidence to be the same in both sexes.

Intussusception has been described in all races.

CAUSATION

Although the cause cannot be definitely stated in each individual case, it is thought that changes in the content of the bowel during weaning on to solid food may be a causative factor in the younger age group.

In older children an intussusception can be due to a cyst or a polyp on the bowel, a Meckel's diverticulum (a small duct abnormally present from embryological days) or haemorrhage into the bowel wall due to some other condition such as leukaemia or Henoch–Schönlein purpura.

In both age groups the cause may be enlargement of specific areas of lymphoid tissue in the bowel as the result of an infective process.

HISTORY

Sir Frederick Treves, in 1898, first described the actual events in the bowel that result in an intussusception. He accurately described the invagination of a part of the bowel into the lumen of another adjacent part. The initial onset of this can be due to any number of factors – as discussed above.

CHARACTERISTICS

Colicky abdominal pain is the first sign of an intussusception. Knees will be drawn up and the baby will become **pale** as the pain heightens. Initially there may be some period of time between these attacks of pain, but as the condition worsens the bouts of colic become more frequent.

Vomiting, due to obstruction of the bowel, will occur following on from this.

Diarrhoea, with the descriptive 'redcurrant' stools, will occur later. Not all babies will show this feature, so diagnosis must not be delayed because of this omission.

A sausage-shaped **swelling** can be felt – in between bouts of colic – usually on the right-hand side of the baby's abdomen or across the top of the abdomen just below the ribs. (This positioning will, of course, vary according to where the intussusception has occurred.)

INVESTIGATIONS

A **plain X-ray** of the abdomen will show where the obstruction is by demonstrating abnormal fluid levels in the bowel.

Ultrasound will also show the position of the intussusception and is usually the preferred investigation.

MANAGEMENT

If the baby is seriously ill and dehydrated, rehydration with **intravenous fluids** will be necessary before any attempt is made to reduce the intussusception. If vomiting has been a prominent feature, a **nasogastric tube** will need to be put in place to remove the contents of the stomach.

Reduction of the intussusception, i.e. the putting back in place of the invaginated bowel (rather like turning an inside-out sleeve right side out), can be done in two ways:

- non-surgically, by the use of a **barium enema** under radiological control. This involves running warm dilute barium into the bowel through a special catheter (with the baby fully sedated). The passage of the barium is watched on the X-ray screen until the position of the intussusception is reached. By the continuing pressure of the column of barium, the invaginated bowel can be pushed back into its normal position. Air, instead of the barium mixture, can also be used successfully to reduce an intussusception. (In China, the air method has been used successfully for centuries – fire-bellows being used to force the air into the bowel!)
- **surgically**, if the non-surgical method has been found to be unsuccessful. The baby is anaesthetized and the intussusception is reduced by hand. Occasionally, a part of the bowel will need to be removed if there is damage. One advantage of the surgical method is that the appendix is usually removed at the same time, which removes the possibility of appendicitis in later life.

THE FUTURE

Very rarely a second intussusception can occur, and this happens whichever method of treatment has been used.

There are no adverse sequelae in later life.

KAWASAKI DISEASE

ALTERNATIVE NAME

Mucocutaneous lymph node syndrome.

INCIDENCE

Kawasaki disease is seen in all parts of the world, but oriental races have the highest incidence. This disease occurs almost exclusively in young children, around 80% of cases being seen in children under the age of 4 years. The end of the first year of life seems to be the most usual time for the condition to occur. It is rarely seen in children over the age of 8 years.

In the UK it is thought that only around 2 children in every 100 000 are affected. Nevertheless, in spite of this being a comparatively rare condition in the UK and the western world, it is vital that the condition is recognized and treated appropriately because of the later complications that can occur.

HISTORY

Kawasaki disease, with over 80 000 reported occurrences, was first described in Japan by Dr Tamisaku Kawasaki about 25 years ago. In Japan epidemics occur, with a 3-year cycle. These epidemics occur more frequently in winter and early spring. This is in distinction to the UK, where no cyclical pattern has been noticed and the disease is seen more often in the spring.

CAUSATION

The cause of Kawasaki disease remains, at present, a mystery. From epidemiological studies and certain features of the disease, the cause would appear to be an infective one. However, even using modern techniques, it has not proved possible to unearth a specific bacterial or viral organism responsible. Work is proceeding on the possibility that a toxin with a specific action on the immune system is the underlying cause.

In spite of Kawasaki disease occurring in epidemics – in Japan at least – there is little evidence of transmission from one child to another. There is also little to suggest that the disease has a genetic basis, although the high susceptibility of oriental children suggests that there may be a racial predisposition to the condition.

CHARACTERISTICS

The characteristics of this unusual, but potentially dangerous, disease are variable. Diagnosis is dependent upon recognition of the clinical signs and symptoms, as there is no specific laboratory test for Kawasaki disease.

Fever is a constant feature and in the early stages of the disease can be the only abnormality. The child's temperature will be high, with spikes of even higher fever. This raised temperature continues for up to 2 weeks, and may continue for a further 2–3 weeks, but as a low-grade fever.

There are a number of other signs and symptoms characterizing Kawasaki disease, and, for a positive diagnosis, at least four of the following conditions need to be present.

- A **rash** appears within 1 week of the onset of the fever, and is very variable in appearance. It can resemble the rash of scarlet fever or that of measles, while at other times the urticarial rash of nettle stings can be seen.
- **Conjunctivitis** – a reddening of the 'white' part of the eye without any obvious pus formation – can be seen soon after the beginning of the fever. As with the fever, this feature can remain for up to 2 weeks.
- **Dryness** and **redness of the lips, tongue and throat** can also occur. Lips can crack and even bleed in severe cases.
- Signs in **fingers and toes** are again a fairly constant sign of Kawasaki disease. Palms of the hands and soles of the feet become reddened and swollen. After around 10–14 days the skin will begin to peel from these extremities.
- **Lymph glands in the neck** are often swollen and tender, although this feature is only seen in about half the children with this disease.

Along with these specific signs and symptoms will be the general irritability and loss of appetite associated with a high temperature, from whatever cause.

It is important that other conditions with somewhat similar symptoms are excluded. These include various bacterial infections of the throat, as well as measles and scarlet fever.

The child will be acutely ill during the initial 2 weeks of the illness. After this time the fever will lessen – although it will frequently still be present – the rash will have disappeared and the lymph nodes subsiding. It is around this time that the skin will be seen to be peeling from hands and feet. At this time also, the child may complain of aching joints.

The most serious aspect of Kawasaki disease is the possible involvement of the **heart and coronary arteries**. This complication is thought to occur in between 20% and 30% of children. Signs of heart and/or coronary artery problems arise within the first 10 days of the illness. **Chest pain** and **pulse irregularities** can occur as well as other signs of heart failure – **breathlessness** and **swollen feet and ankles**. These difficulties generally resolve with appropriate treatment. Occasionally, however, permanent damage can be done to the coronary arteries with the formation of an aneurysm (a balloon-ing) in one of the tiny blood vessels that supply the heart muscle with vital oxygen. This aneurysm can rupture, or the heart muscle be so starved of oxygen that a 'heart attack' is the fatal outcome. This tragic scenario is uncommon, but must always be remembered as a remote possibility.

INVESTIGATIONS

Blood tests give useful, but unspecific, information. There is often an asso-ciated abnormality in the platelets – the part of the blood concerned with the regulation of clotting mechanisms.

Echocardiography is advisable when the diagnosis of Kawasaki disease is certain. This will show up any heart involvement that has occurred and should be repeated 6 weeks after the onset of the illness.

MANAGEMENT

Aspirin is the mainstay of treatment in Kawasaki disease. It acts by lower-ing temperature and helps prevent the platelets in the blood from clump-ing together. (Aspirin is usually not recommended for children under the age of 12 years. This is because of the possibility of Reye's syndrome, in which it is thought aspirin in some children may play a part. But with Kawasaki disease the benefits of aspirin in preventing heart damage outweigh this remote risk.)

High doses of aspirin are necessary for the first week of the disease. A lower dose of aspirin is then given until around 6 weeks after the onset of the disease, when heart damage – monitored by echocardiography – is eliminated.

Gammaglobulin given intravenously has been used in clinical trials in the USA and Japan and has been shown to lessen the risk of heart involve-ment. This treatment is generally reserved for children who already have some form of heart disease or those children who are at high risk of heart involvement, most usually babies under the age of 1 year with a severe attack of Kawasaki disease.

A further drug as an alternative to aspirin or gammaglobulin can be used that acts successfully on the platelets. The appropriate treatment will need to be decided for each individual child.

General nursing care with sufficient **rest**, a **light diet** and **plenty of flu-ids** will also be needed during the acute phase of the illness. Also a suffi-ciently **long convalescent period** is necessary for it to be certain that there has been no heart damage.

THE FUTURE

This will obviously depend on whether or not heart involvement has oc-curred. Without this complication, there are no known after-effects from an attack of Kawasaki disease.

SELF-HELP GROUP

Kawasaki Support Group
13 Norwood Grove
Potters Green
Coventry, CV2 2FR
Tel. 01203 612178.

LICE

ALTERNATIVE NAME

Nits. (This is not a true alternative name, as the 'nits' are the eggs of the louse, but in common parlance – in the UK at least – many people refer to lice by this colloquial name.)

INCIDENCE

There are three types of human louse – the head louse, the body louse and the 'crab' or pubic louse. The first two are similar but merely affect different parts of the body – as evidenced by the name. The pubic louse is a different, quite distinct species.

Lice occur worldwide, and are especially prominent in areas with low standards of hygiene. The head louse is the one most commonly seen in the UK and will be the type described.

The incidence of the head louse varies enormously from place to place and from time to time with no obvious explanation for these facts. During an 'epidemic' of infestation with the head louse as many as 60% of children in schools can be affected at any one time. A survey carried out in 1977 estimated that around 200 000 children in England were infected with head lice – a sizeable problem.

Infestation is commonest in the 3–13-year-old age group – the incidence peaking among the 6–9-year-olds. Girls seem to be more commonly affected than boys. Strangely enough, hair length seems to have little bearing on whether lice are present or not. Both clean and dirty heads can be infested.

CAUSATION

Infestation is with the head louse. Although the head is most frequently and most heavily infested, other hairy parts of the body can also be involved.

The insects live close to the roots of the hair, and feed on blood, which they suck from the underlying skin. The female lays around six to eight eggs ('nits') every 24 hours. These nits are stuck firmly to the shafts of hair close to the scalp initially. (Obviously as the hair grows, so the nits will be found lower down the shaft away from the head.) These hatch within about 10 days, and so the cycle is repeated, unless treatment to eradicate the lice – and the eggs – is given. The female louse lives for about a month. So in this time around 240 eggs can be laid!

CHARACTERISTICS

There may be **no symptoms at all** in a child with a minimal number of head lice. The first clue as to an infestation may be parents or school teachers seeing the characteristic white nits on the hair shafts.

Under conditions where there is a heavy infestation the child's head may **itch**. This irritation is probably due to an allergic reaction to the presence of the louse and not to the movement of the insect. Any child who is continually scratching his/her head should be examined closely for the presence of lice. There are few other conditions in which there is such obvious irritation of the scalp alone. The most common places for the lice to congregate are behind the ears and on the back of the head.

The itching of the scalp can cause the child to be a **restless sleeper**, because of the constant low-grade irritation.

Excessive scratching of the scalp can cause an **infection** of the skin, giving rise to impetigo. This can cause a mild **fever** and, in severe cases, enlargement of the **glands in the neck**. So any child with a mild fever and tender, swollen neck glands, but with no sore throat or other 'coldy' symptoms should have the head examined for head lice. If impetigo has occurred because of excessive scratching, antibiotic treatment will be required.

Transmission of the head louse is by head-to-head contact. This, of course, is a very common event among small children, who frequently have their heads close together during play or during school activities. It is also thought that the lice can be passed on by the sharing of hair brushes and combs or by merely trying on the hat or other headgear of an infested playmate. Obviously, situations where there is overcrowding of children provide excellent conditions for the head louse to infect a number of children.

MANAGEMENT

On discovery of an infestation in one child, the whole class – including the teaching staff – should have their heads examined for lice. In the UK, the school health service usually undertakes this task when contacted by parents or teachers. (A decade or so ago, regular head inspections were all part of the routine health care in schools. This has now been suspended because of the professional time consumed for little apparent result. Control has been found to be better achieved by call-out when necessary.)

There are a number of preparations (**lotions and shampoos**) that effectively kill the head louse. The type used has to be changed in any one area at fairly frequent intervals because of the rapidity with which the louse becomes resistant to any one preparation. Good liaison between health authorities is necessary to preserve the efficacy of the preparations used.

The lotion or shampoo is applied to the child's head in the evening, allowed to dry naturally, and combed out the following morning. (The lotion is probably preferable to the shampoo.) This one treatment should effectively kill all the lice. But the nits can remain stuck to the shafts of the hair and may need combing out using a fine-toothed nit comb. Success has also been achieved simply by **frequent combing with a fine-toothed comb** for a minimum of **10 days**. This must be done conscientiously on a regular basis, but taking care not to make the child's head sore by overzealous combing.

There is no need to exclude the child from **school** once the treatment has been given. **Every family member,** including grandparents, should have the lotion applied to his/her hair once one child in the family is found to be infested – even if no lice or nits are found on other children or parents. This will ensure that no minute, lurking louse will survive. (Care must be taken that the lotion does not splash into the child's eyes, as it will cause severe irritation. Also, of course, care must be taken with the storage of the lotion – accidental ingestion by a toddler will need emergency treatment.)

PREVENTION

- Rapid and adequate **treatment of the whole family** once an infested member is found is the best way of prevention once an initial child is infected.
- Advise children not to borrow each other's **hats, combs,** etc.
- Advise parents on **adequate and frequent brushing, combing** and **washing** of children's hair.

Much emotion and upset can be caused by infestation with head lice in a school. But it must be remembered that, once the lice are present in a class, they can just as easily pass to a beautifully clean head as to a less desirable one!

LIMP

The incidence of limps in children can only be classified as part of that of the various conditions for which this symptom is an important part. It is, however, vital that any child who limps for any significant period of time should be fully investigated.

CAUSATION

The causes of a limp in children can range from the trivial, such as a blister or a verruca somewhere on the foot, to the serious, such as a septic arthritis or a tumour.

Signs and symptoms, with subsequent investigations and treatment, are related to the causative factor.

Conditions in the feet

Conditions such as verrucas, blisters or a minor fracture following injury can cause a child to limp.

Blisters will need cleaning gently, but with no attempt to burst the blister if the skin is still intact. A simple Elastoplast dressing with removal of the offending footwear is all the treatment that is necessary. (If the covering skin is removed from a blister – either accidentally or on purpose – exposing raw tissue, cellulitis can result. This inflammation of the connective tissues around the wound can spread alarmingly and affect the whole leg. Appropriate and rapid antibiotic treatment is necessary under these conditions.)

Verrucas are a particularly common finding in the 11–16-year-old age group, and can cause sufficient pain as to cause a limp at times. (This condition is dealt with under Warts.)

Fractures of the small bones of the foot can occur, sometimes after a seemingly minor injury. If the child describes either a crushing or a twisting injury, and is still in pain a day or two after the event, medical advice should be sought. An X-ray will confirm or exclude this cause for a limp.

Foreign bodies in the foot are a common hazard of childhood, especially following barefoot physical exercise. Children will readily be able to point to the site of the implanted object. Removal will give relief and a return to a normal gait.

One of the **osteochondrites** (see under Perthes' disease, below) can affect the foot, causing a child to limp. Sever's disease is an osteochondritis of the heel, while Kohler's disease is a similar problem affecting one of the tiny bones of the foot. The typical picture of osteochondritis can be seen on X-ray. Immobilization in plaster for 6–8 weeks may be necessary, although many milder cases will settle with a reduction in activity.

Juvenile chronic arthritis can first be manifest in the ankles. The child will complain of pain, and can limp in an endeavour to relieve this. This can be one of the first signs of the poly- or pauciarticular types of juvenile arthritis (see under Arthritis, above).

Conditions in the hip

Perthes' disease is a further example of one of the osteochondrites – this time affecting the hip. A limp can be the only sign of this condition for some time.

A **slipped femoral epiphysis** can be a further cause of a limp in an older child – usually in the early adolescent years. In this condition the growing head of the femur gradually slips until it is in a non-aligned position in relation to the pelvic bone. Occasionally the condition can occur suddenly as a result of a twisting injury. Under these circumstances the pain is acute and the child will be unable to move the affected leg. Boys are slightly more often affected than girls. Overweight children are thought to be more at risk from a slipped femoral epiphysis.

As well as a limp, the young person is most likely to complain of pain in the knee – although the problem is in the hip. (Diseases of the hip often manifest themselves with pain referred to the knee joint. So any investigation of knee pain should include close examination of the hips.) On examination, there is swelling and limitation of the affected hip. X-ray examination will confirm the diagnosis. Operative procedures are necessary to realign the head of the femur in the pelvis.

'Irritable hip' (transient synovitis) is a relatively common condition arising out of the blue with no known specific causative factor. The child will limp, and the muscles around the hip joint will be found to be in spasm. There may be an associated mild fever. Blood tests may also show a raised erythrocyte sedimentation rate (ESR). This condition usually settles adequately and quickly with a short period of bed rest.

Miscellaneous conditions

One of the most potentially disabling causes of a long-term limp is an undiagnosed (in babyhood) **congenital dislocation of the hip**. Fortunately, this is a rare occurrence in the UK today, where the hips of all babies are routinely examined at birth and at subsequent progress checks. But the possibility of this condition must always be remembered, particularly if the child has been born in a part of the world where such checks are not routinely performed.

Certain other – rare – conditions in which there is an **inequality in leg length** can cause a limp. This includes a congenitally shortened bone in a leg, or a scoliosis (a sideways twist in the spine due to a variety of causes). An attack of poliomyelitis can cause a shortening of one leg – again a rare cause these days in the developed countries, but still to be remembered in a child who has lived in a country where poliomyelitis is still endemic.

The possibility of a **tumour** – benign or malignant – in one of the leg bones must also be considered. Pain and swelling over the site are the most usual manifestations, but a limp can also be one of the first signs in a younger child. Further investigations, followed by appropriate treatment, must be instigated rapidly if a tumour is suspected.

Finally, the possibility of **non-accidental injury** must always be considered in a child with a limp. Careful examination of the whole of the child's body must be undertaken, with follow-up X-rays if necessary, to exclude injuries for which there is no rational explanation.

Most limps in children are due to trivial and obvious causes. But important and treatable diseases can be missed if a long-term limp is ignored.

Measles

Alternative name

Rubeola.

Incidence

Notification of this disease began in 1940, and the number of cases reported was high in the decades up to the mid-1960s. It was at this time that immunization against measles was introduced. As many as 800 000 children every year suffered from this infection before the advent of immunization, and the incidence of the disease showed a marked biennial variation – every other year being a 'bad' measles year.

Since the introduction of the measles vaccine in the mid-1960s, the incidence of the infection has fallen dramatically, in the 1970s and 1980s averaging around 100 000 notifications or fewer every year.

In 1988 the MMR (measles, mumps and rubella) vaccine was introduced and is now given routinely to all babies between the first and second years of life. Since this time, the notification of cases of measles has dropped to the low hundreds every year.

Measles occurs most frequently in the 5–10-year-old age group, although in crowded urban conditions younger children contract the infection. Measles is extremely rare under the age of 6 months. Antibodies from the mother protect the baby from the infection during these critical early months of life.

In developing countries, who have not the benefit of the measles vaccine and in whose children malnutrition is an ever-present problem, measles is a potent killer. As many as 25% of children die from this infection.

Although measles, as with many of the other so-called 'childhood' infections, is comparatively mild today, complications can – and do – still occur. There are, regretfully, still a few deaths in the UK every year attributable to measles. Children who have other serious conditions, such as leukaemia, are especially at risk.

History

In some parts of rural Africa today, babies are not given a name until the expected measles epidemic has passed. The death rate is so high among young children that parents feel that they cannot risk positively identifying their child until he or she has successfully survived the measles epidemic.

Causation

Measles is caused by a virus and is a highly infectious condition. Transmission is by droplet infection from the respiratory tract. The infection is usually passed on before the typical rash appears, and hence before a definite diagnosis of measles is made.

The incubation period is between 8 and 14 days.

Characteristics

Measles begins in much the same way as does any common cold, namely:

- a **runny nose**, associated with catarrhal symptoms;
- **sore, inflamed eyes** with marked photophobia (a dislike of light);
- a harsh, dry **cough**;
- a **fever** of varying degree;
- general **malaise**;
- **convulsions** sometimes occur as a result of the high fever.

These are all very generalized symptoms, which can initially be thought to be due to a number of causes, e.g. the current upper respiratory tract infection that is 'going the rounds'. But, within 2 or 3 days a very specific sign of measles can be noted in the child's mouth. Small white spots, which have been likened to grains of salt, appear on the insides of the cheeks opposite the back teeth. These are known as **Koplik spots** and only occur with an infection with the measles virus.

On the third or fourth day of the illness the diagnosis becomes obvious with the appearance of the typical **rash**. This starts behind the ears and along the hair-line. It spreads rapidly to involve the whole body and limbs – the face and upper chest being usually most involved. The dusky red spots coalesce, giving rise to a blotchy appearance.

The rash begins to fade after 3 or 4 days, often with some shedding of the surface skin. (This is rather like the desquamation seen in scarlet fever. In measles, however, the hands and feet are not involved.)

With the appearance of the rash, a **high fever** can recur. This will improve as the rash fades. In uncomplicated cases of measles, improvement is rapid following the disappearance of the rash, and within a week, in mild cases, the child will be returned to full health. Occasionally the dry cough will persist for a week or two.

Investigations

These are rarely, if ever, needed to make a diagnosis of measles, as the signs and symptoms are so definite once the rash has appeared. The virus can be isolated and grown from the secretions of the nose and throat as well as the urine of a sufferer.

COMPLICATIONS

It is the complications that can occur with measles that make this infection so potentially dangerous. For descriptive purposes, it is convenient to look at these in relationship to the body system involved.

Respiratory tract

There is always an associated respiratory involvement with an attack of measles. The trachea (windpipe), larynx and bronchi are all involved in this viral infection, as is evidenced by the sore throat and dry cough. Secondary infection with bacteria is an ever-real threat when these tissues are damaged by the measles virus. Bronchitis is almost an inevitable accompaniment to measles and pneumonia a common complication.

Symptoms of further involvement of the respiratory tract will include:

- a **return of fever**;
- a **worsening of the cough**.

Further medical advice should always be sought if these symptoms should occur in a child who is getting over an attack of measles. Antibiotics, and perhaps hospital admission, will be necessary under these circumstances.

Central nervous system

Convulsions can occur during the early stages of the infection. Medical advice should always be sought for a child who has had a convulsion.

Encephalitis (inflammation of the brain) is the most serious complication of measles. The time at which signs and symptoms appear can vary, but most usually they occur around 7–10 days after the beginning of the illness. The child will become **drowsy**, suffer from **convulsions** and have a return of the **fever**. Specific neurological signs may also occur, such as weakening or paralysis of a limb. This serious state of affairs can either:

- show a steady slow improvement with no permanent after-effects;
- show a slow recovery, but leave the child with permanent neurological and/or intellectual damage;
- show a steady deterioration resulting in a fatal outcome.

A rare form of encephalitis can occur some 5–10 years after an attack of measles. This is known as 'subacute sclerosing panencephalitis' and is an extremely serious condition. The child shows at first some falling-off of intellectual abilities, together with some instability of posture and difficulty in movement. This vicious condition progresses inexorably into paralysis and dementia and finally coma and death. This condition is thought to be due to a reactivation, by some unknown stimulus, of the measles virus, which has remained latent in the brain.

Eyes

The conjunctiva of the eye is involved to some degree in every case of measles as is evidenced by the **photophobia** complained of by most children with measles.

As with the respiratory tract, secondary bacterial infection can result in **irritation of the cornea**.

Ears

Otitis media used to be an almost invariable accompaniment to measles. Earache and high fever with possible rupture of the eardrum and/or mastoiditis added to the miseries of the child with measles. Fortunately, today, because of the apparently lower virulence of the measles virus as well as prompt antibiotic treatment, this is an unusual complication.

Gastrointestinal tract

The whole of the gut seems to be involved in the measles infection, ranging from soreness in the mouth to indigestion and abdominal pain. As well as direct involvement of the gut in the generalized infection, lymph glands in the abdomen are also enlarged by the infective process – yet one further uncomfortable and unpleasant aspect of this viral disease.

MANAGEMENT

This will obviously be different for the child with complications from the child suffering from an uncomplicated attack of measles.

Uncomplicated measles

Adequate rest is necessary, **in bed** during the initial stages of the infection if symptoms are at all severe. When the child's temperature has settled and energy is returning, quiet play in a warm room is satisfactory.

An **adequate fluid intake** is necessary to ensure that the child does not become dehydrated. High fever causes fluid loss through perspiration – and unwillingness to eat and drink also causes dehydration. Food should not be forced on the child, but plenty of drinks – of any kind – should be encouraged.

Paracetamol, in any form in appropriate dosage, will help to lower temperature as well as relieving headache and sore throat.

While a **darkened room** will not in any way improve the sore eyes so commonly associated with measles, the child will probably feel more comfortable in subdued light. Soothing eye-drops can also be prescribed.

Antibiotics have no part to play in an uncomplicated attack of measles. (These drugs are not active against viral infections.) But if there is any suggestion of secondary bacterial infection anywhere in the body, antibiotics should be prescribed.

Complicated attack of measles

Antibiotics, usually penicillin, will be needed if respiratory or ear involvement occurs.

Neurological involvement will usually necessitate **admission to hospital** for nursing, monitoring and an adequate nutrition programme.

Long-term management of the results of complications of measles will depend on how much permanent damage has been done. **Neurological** and/or **intellectual problems** will need **regular review** for many months, as improvement can be maintained for some time after the initial infection has subsided. Intellectual abilities will also need regular assessment and review, with special schooling arranged if necessary. **Hearing** should be checked a month or so after full recovery if the ears have been involved to any degree. Children can be left with varying degrees of deafness after measles, and it is important that this is recognized and appropriate help given.

Measles is an unpleasant disease with potent serious complications, and should never be taken lightly. Fortunately, with the advent of immunization against the disease the incidence has reduced dramatically. Nevertheless, measles does still occur and will continue to do so until at least 90% of children have benefited from the vaccine. Even mild cases can leave a child debilitated. It is wise to avoid too many active pursuits for a week or two after recovery, and to ensure that the convalescent child receives adequate rest and nutrition.

PREVENTION

Prevention is by **immunization**. This is done routinely in the UK today at between 1 and 2 years of age by the **MMR** vaccine. (A booster at 4 to 5 years of age is also given.) This vaccine should be given even if the child has been thought to have had an attack of naturally occurring measles previously. Age is no bar to receiving this vaccine if it has been missed at the usual time.

Contraindications to receiving the vaccine are the usual ones of:

- an acute feverish illness at the time when the immunization is due – the vaccine should be given when the child has recovered;
- children with any form of malignant disease or those receiving immunosuppressant drugs for any reason.

Allergy to eggs at one time caused much alarm among mothers, and many children were denied the benefits of the vaccine merely because they disliked eggs. The only reason for not giving the vaccine in this context is if the child has a **severe reaction when eating eggs** – such as swelling of the mouth and throat or difficulty in breathing.

THE FUTURE

An attack of measles confers immunity for life. Apart from the rare possibility of subacute sclerosing panencephalitis, neurological or hearing damage from one of the complications, there are no other adverse effects in later life from an attack of measles.

When immunization levels of children have reached the advised target, measles should be an infection of the past as is, for example, poliomyelitis today. But meanwhile children can still suffer from measles. It must also be remembered that measles is still a common, and much-feared, disease in developing countries and, with today's ease of travel, unimmunized people are at risk of acquiring the infection.

Meningitis

Incidence

Meningitis is caused by a wide variety of viruses and bacteria. The viruses that can cause meningitis are numerous and so the exact incidence of cases of viral meningitis is difficult to classify.

Bacterial meningitis also has a large number of responsible bacteria (see below). Figures for meningococcal meningitis (caused by the bacterium *Neisseria meningitidis*) are well-documented and the illness due to this cause can be seen to occur in peaks. For example, in the early 1970s over 1000 cases were notified. In the early 1980s this figure fell to around 400, but in the late 1980s notifications were again as high as 1300 cases.

Meningitis due to bacteria is essentially an infection of childhood, and over 80% of all notified cases are in children under the age of 15 years. A high majority of these occur in children under the age of 5 years.

Causation

The **viruses** capable of causing meningitis are multiple. They range from such viruses as those causing measles and mumps through the common Echo- and Coxsackie viruses to other specific viruses, such as Herpes simplex and Epstein–Barr virus. A formidable list!

Bacteria capable of causing meningitis are less numerous, but still not an inconsiderable number. In the early days of life, meningitis is more often due to infection with certain types of *Streptococcus, E. coli* and the *Haemophilus influenzae* type b bacterium. *Haemophilus influenzae* b (Hib) is the commonest cause of meningitis in the 1–4-year-old age group.

Characteristics

Whatever the infecting agent causing the illness, the characteristics (with a few exceptions) are similar.

- **Headache** and/or **pain at the back of the neck** is one of the most frequent early features. Associated with the pain at the back of the neck is a reluctance to bend the head forward. For example, if the child is asked to 'kiss the knees' it is impossible to do so without an exacerbation of the pain in the back of the neck.
- **Nausea and vomiting** – unassociated with abdominal pain – is also a common feature. The vomiting can be projectile in character.
- **Fever** of varying degree is the usual accompaniment to these symptoms.

- **Photophobia** (a dislike of light) can be marked, with the child turning away from the window and burying his/her face in the pillow.
- **Drowsiness and irritability** on being disturbed can occur within a few hours.
- **Convulsions** can also occur.
- With a specific type of meningitis – meningococcal meningitis – there is an associated **rash**. This is very specific, and consists of numerous, small, bruise-like spots all over the body, which do not fade on pressure. This is a sign of a serious infection that can be rapidly fatal – within hours – unless treatment is given.

In younger children, under 2 years, these characteristic signs are not so well marked. **Fever, vomiting** and **pallor**, together with a **high-pitched cry** and **refusal of feeds**, can be all that is noticed initially. **Drowsiness** and/or **convulsions** are later serious signs in these younger children.

INVESTIGATIONS

A **lumbar puncture** to obtain cerebrospinal fluid must be performed, in hospital, before treatment is started. (There is one major exception to this. If meningococcal meningitis is suspected – the specific rash being a strong diagnostic feature – immediate treatment with intramuscular penicillin must be given before removal to hospital.) The cerebrospinal fluid thus obtained is seen to be cloudy in cases of meningitis. Laboratory examination will be able to determine the infecting agent.

Blood tests to determine the infecting agent are also useful.

MANAGEMENT

The child with meningitis can be seriously ill, and will often require to be admitted to hospital for treatment.

- **Antibiotic** treatment is begun immediately after the cerebrospinal fluid has been obtained by lumbar puncture. (The reason why treatment is not started before this investigation is done – except, of course, in the case of suspected meningococcal meningitis – is that treatment can confuse the laboratory diagnosis as to which infecting agent is present.) Penicillin and/or chloramphenicol are the most usual antibiotics used, and it is usual to continue to give these drugs for at least 10 days.
- **Fluids**, intravenously initially, can be necessary. The young child can become rapidly dehydrated if vomiting and fever are severe. Refusal to eat or drink also results in lack of fluid in the body.

Regular **monitoring** of the child's temperature, pulse, respiration and level of consciousness is also an important necessity. If there is any deterioration shown by these regular readings immediate help can be given.

If convulsions have occurred, or if the child is extremely restless, **anticonvulsant drugs** may be necessary for a short while.

Parents will need **emotional support** and perhaps also **physical help** (with other children or with travelling to hospital, for example) during their child's serious illness.

With an uncomplicated attack of meningitis, recovery is complete with no permanent after-effects. Following discharge from hospital, it is wise to allow the child a week or two's convalescence before returning to the rough and tumble of the school day. Extra rest and a nutritious diet will help to restore general health following this serious illness.

COMPLICATIONS

Serious long-term complications can occur following a severe attack of meningitis. Probably the most common complication is **sensorineural deafness**. From studies on the complications of meningitis, around 10% of children are found to have some degree of deafness following meningitis. This appears to depend very much on the organism causing the infection. Infection with *Streptococcus* was shown in one study to affect 30% of the children suffering from this type of meningitis.

All children should have their hearing tested a month or two after recovery from meningitis. Hearing aids and/or special schooling may be needed with the more severe cases. It is important that good liaison is maintained between health and education authorities involved with these children.

Epilepsy can be a late complication of meningitis. There does not appear to be any correlation between later epilepsy and the type of infecting organism. Children who have had convulsions during the initial stages of their illness are most likely to develop later epilepsy. It is thought that this complication affects around 5% of children following meningitis.

Anticonvulsant drugs will be necessary to control seizures.

Mental retardation can regretfully be a sequel to meningitis. The child's abilities (at school if a school-age child) will be seen to have fallen off since the illness. In preschool children, skills previously learned may be lost, and only regained slowly. Regular developmental checks are necessary for the preschool child to determine the extent of the damage. These should be repeated regularly over succeeding months, as recovery can continue for some time after the acute stage of the illness is over. Again, special educational facilities may be required, with close liaison between health and education authorities.

Cerebral palsy, in which there are problems with control of the muscles of the body, can also occur after an attack of meningitis. Limbs can either become stiff and rigid with much difficulty in walking, or floppy and weak. Here again, regular assessment by a paediatrician skilled in handicapping motor conditions is vital. Physiotherapy is also important to enable the child to make the most of his/her residual abilities.

Speech problems may be also part of the picture, and help from a speech therapist is invaluable under these circumstances.

Mental retardation may also be an associated handicap, although this is not invariably so. Mental handicap and/or cerebral palsy are thought to affect 3–8% of children following an attack of meningitis.

PREVENTION

One form of meningitis is now preventable by **immunization**. This is the meningitis due to the *Haemophilus influenzae* type b bacterium – the most common type of meningitis seen in children between the ages of 1 and 4 years.

Immunization with this vaccine is part of the routine babyhood immunization schedule in the UK. Three injections of the vaccine, at monthly intervals, are given at the same time as the triple vaccine (against diphtheria, tetanus and whooping-cough) at 2, 3 and 4 months of age. This affords protection for the child over the years when infection with this type of organism is at its height. Work is progressing on combining this vaccine with the triple vaccine.

There are no contraindications to a baby receiving this vaccine, apart from the usual ones of an acute illness (when the immunization should be postponed) or where there has been a severe reaction to a previous dose of vaccine. These reactions are virtually unknown. No serious reaction has been reported after the giving of over 20 million doses of this vaccine. Minor reactions, such as redness and swelling around the injection site for a few hours, do occur, but resolve rapidly.

There are no vaccines, or other preventive methods, against meningitis due to other infection organisms.

Outbreaks of meningococcal meningitis in nurseries or schools will need public health advice as to the advisability of giving penicillin, or vaccine, to children in close contact with the sufferer from this form of meningitis.

THE FUTURE

Following an attack of meningitis in childhood, there are no deleterious after-effects unless complications – as discussed above – have occurred. These, of course, can be severe, needing long-term specialized help.

SELF-HELP GROUP

National Meningitis Trust
Fern House
Bath Road
Stroud
Gloucester, GL5 3TJ
Tel. 01454 281 811
    0808 800 3344 (help line)
Fax 01454 281 094.

MIGRAINE

INCIDENCE

Migraine is rare under the age of 2 years. The incidence of this unpleasant condition increases with age until, by school age, around 50 children in every 1000 are thought to have suffered from an attack of migraine at one time or another.

Before puberty the number of boys suffering from migraine is about twice the number of girls. At puberty, however, the number of male sufferers decreases and that in females increases until the adult incidence of excess attacks in women is reached. This indicates that the alteration in incidence must bear some relationship to hormonal changes at around the time of puberty.

HISTORY

Socrates gave accounts of classic migraine around 25 centuries ago, so migraine is certainly not a new environmental disease! Lewis Carroll of *Alice in Wonderland* fame was known to suffer from severe attacks of migraine. Hallucinations of becoming smaller and smaller – so graphically described in his story – are typical of a certain specific late effect of migraine.

CAUSATION

Migraine is thought to be due to alterations in the reactions of the blood-vessels supplying the brain. There is a phase when these vessels constrict and become smaller and so reduce the blood flow to the particular part of the brain supplied. A subsequent phase occurs when the vessels dilate and the blood supply is increased. Different blood vessels can be affected at different times. This probably accounts for the wide variety of symptoms seen in this condition.

These effects on the blood vessels are due in turn to a wide variety of stimuli. These range from genetic susceptibility through reaction to certain foods and exercise to possible hormonal imbalance and reaction to viral infections.

Genetic predisposition

It has been found that 90% of children suffering from migraine have one or more members of the immediate family who also suffer from this condition.

Food

Foods that are most often implicated in the onset of an attack of migraine are **cheese** and **chocolate**, with **oranges** a close third. The two former foods contain a substance, tyramine, which is a powerful dilator of blood vessels.

Monosodium glutamate has also been blamed, and may be the cause of attacks of migraine from which some people suffer after eating a Chinese meal. This substance, a flavour-enhancer, is an ingredient in many – delicious – Chinese menus.

Milk products, eggs and **gluten-containing foods** (gluten being the product found in wheat and wheat products) have at times also been considered to precipitate attacks of migraine. These foods may also precipitate other conditions (such as coeliac disease, which results from an allergy to gluten) and the migraine may be but one symptom of a generalized food intolerance.

Other causes

Exercise, particularly if associated with competitive sports, may precipitate migraine in some children. It can be difficult to decide whether it is the exercise itself or the worry of the competition that causes the problem! (Again, under these circumstances, true migraine can easily be confused with the so-called 'tension' headaches, although these are rare before adolescence.)

Sex hormones, androgens and oestrogens, are probably responsible for the change in incidence of migraine seen at puberty. The extra androgens secreted by boys around the time of puberty appear to reduce the tendency to migraine, while oestrogens in higher levels in girls after puberty appear to increase the tendency. Changes in oestrogen levels at various times in the menstrual cycle also influence the timing of attacks in some girls.

It is possible that a **viral infection** can precipitate an attack of migraine in a susceptible individual. This may be difficult to differentiate from the headache due to the infection itself in children. (With age and experience, the person suffering from migraine will be only too well aware of the difference!)

Having listed the possible causes, it is no wonder that migraine is so difficult to control.

CHARACTERISTICS

Migraine, for descriptive purposes, can be divided into a number of subtypes – each caused by changes in the blood vessels but with slightly differing symptoms.

Classical migraine has a very definite 'aura' followed by a one-sided headache. This aura usually takes the form of visual manifestations, but specific smells have also been described. The visual aura can consist, for example, of blurring of the vision or flashes of light compounded by a zig-zag pattern. Also, some people experience an absence of part of their visual field, leaving words and sentences chopped in half. These visual effects are found in around 30% of children with migraine, and can be very worrying to the child when they are first experienced. The headache usually follows on after the visual manifestations or they can arise together.

Common migraine is less likely to be associated with an aura. The headache is also not so likely to be felt on one side of the head, but more as a generalized headache. Nausea and/or vomiting can accompany this type of migraine as well as general feelings of malaise.

Complicated migraine is said to occur when attacks of giddiness and/or periodic attacks of vomiting ('cyclical vomiting' or 'abdominal migraine') occur. The headache under these circumstances is not the most prominent feature. Children with this type of cyclical vomiting – which can also be accompanied by abdominal pain – frequently go on to develop the more usual forms of migraine in later life.

It can be difficult to differentiate the attacks of giddiness from epilepsy, as the child can be so dizzy as to fall to the ground during an attack.

Children with any form of migraine also appear to suffer from travel sickness more frequently than do other children – the figure quoted is about 40%.

INVESTIGATIONS

It is important, before settling on a diagnosis of migraine, that other physical causes for the headache are excluded. Other serious conditions that could be the cause of the headache in children are brain tumours, continued bleeding into the brain following even a mild head injury, raised blood pressure or a previously undiagnosed hydrocephalus (an excess of fluid in specialized cavities of the brain.)

As a brief guide, any child with a combination of:

- a headache that is **worse on waking** from sleep;
- a headache that **wakes him/her** from sleep;
- a headache that is **worse on coughing**;
- persistent **visual problems** – such as seeing coloured lights or zigzag lines for several days;
- a **behaviour change** for no obvious reason;
- **neurological symptoms**, such as weakness of any part of the body;
- **no family history** of migraine;

should be further investigated to find the reason for the headaches. (Other less serious causes, such as sinusitis, should also be excluded before a diagnosis of migraine is arrived at.)

Investigations under these circumstances include:

- checking on the **blood pressure** after a careful history of the type and timing of the headaches has been taken;
- an **electroencephalogram**, especially if the child becomes drowsy or confused in association with the headaches.

- a **CT scan** if symptoms suggest that the headaches may be due to a serious and treatable cause.

If none of the pointers suggests a cause other than migraine, a few simple investigations will help to identify 'triggering' factors:

- **relationship to stressful events** – even such enjoyable ones as birthday parties or theatre visits as well as the more obvious ones, such as competitive sports or exams of any kind;
- discussion with school teachers regarding the child's **progress in school** – worries about difficulties in certain areas of schooling may be causing the child frustration that is showing itself by headaches.

MANAGEMENT

Many of the migraine attacks suffered by both children and adults can be aborted by **lying down** in a darkened, quiet room for an hour. This is most frequently successful if this action is taken before the attack is fully developed. Children who are used to attacks of migraine will know when an attack is imminent. Sympathetic parents and/or teachers (particularly those who suffer from migraine themselves) will encourage the child to lie down as soon as symptoms become obvious.

Analgesics, such as paracetamol compounds, will also shorten an attack if taken early enough, particularly if combined with a period of rest.

Antiemetic drugs, such as stemetil, are useful if nausea and vomiting are a problem. Again, if they are taken at the first warning signs of an attack, the effect can be greater.

Children with 'cyclical vomiting' – a special type of complicated migraine – can benefit from regular treatment with one of the antiemetic drugs. This can be especially helpful during a period of stress when attacks of vomiting and/or headache occur with monotonous regularity.

Drugs acting directly on the blood vessels are also available. Their use in children, however, is limited, both because of the type of migraine commonly suffered by children and because of the side-effects of these drugs. Only in intractable migraine, and then under strict medical supervision, are these drugs used.

Biofeedback techniques have been tried with some children, with varying degrees of success. Here, measurement of the skin resistance and blood-flow followed by techniques to alter this are used.

Elimination diets can also be tried for children in whom other methods have failed and where there is thought to be a food component.

Common-sense handling of the attacks by all adults involved with the child is also of importance. Too much emphasis on the migraine will cause concern, and hence further attacks. The difficult balancing act between sympathetic understanding and encouragement is an art to be learned by all parents of children who suffer from migraine.

Prevention

Choosing to be born into a family who have no idea of what a migrainous headache is like is probably the best – but completely unattainable! – way to prevent migraine. **Avoidance of foods** that are known to bring on an attack is also an obvious way of prevention.

Stressful situations can to a certain extent be controlled as the child matures and becomes more in control of both environment and stressful situations. Checking on the possibility of learning difficulties, with **remedial teaching** made available if this is positive, can do much to relieve the stress of repeated failure.

The future

Migraine fortunately tends to decrease both in frequency and severity with age, but this may not occur until early middle age has been reached. The teenage years and the 20s and 30s can be trying, but experience will show how best to avoid or abort attacks.

Mumps

Alternative name

Epidemic parotitis.

Incidence

Until 1988, mumps was not a notifiable disease in the UK, so accurate figures on the number of children contracting the disease are not available. Hospital records show, however, that about 1200 admissions to hospital each year in England and Wales were due to mumps or to one of the complications of the infection.

Children of both sexes between the ages of 5 and 15 years are the usual sufferers from an attack of mumps. It is rare in children below the age of 5 years.

History

Mumps has been mentioned historically for many years. In fact, 'mump' is an old English word meaning 'mope' – a good description of someone with the uncomfortably swollen face of mumps!

Causation

Mumps is an infectious disease of the salivary glands caused by a specific virus. The parotid salivary glands situated on each side of the face below and in front of the ears are the glands most commonly – and obviously – affected. The other salivary glands, beneath the chin and tongue, are also frequently affected.

The condition is spread by droplet infection from the breath of a sufferer. Children are infectious for several days before the obvious signs of mumps appear. The incubation period of the disease is 14–21 days. The infection can be passed on for several days after the swelling of the glands becomes apparent.

Immunity to the virus is lifelong following an attack of mumps.

Characteristics

As with many of the infectious 'childhood' fevers, mumps can begin with the very general symptoms of **headache, fever, loss of appetite** and a general feeling of ill-health – all very non-specific. But within 2–3 days, the diagnosis will become obvious when **pain and swelling in the parotid glands** (and maybe the other salivary glands as well) occurs. Occasionally this swelling can be the first sign of the condition, the usual prodromal symptoms being absent. Either one or both of the parotid glands can be involved. The swellings may be small or very large and extremely painful and tender. Sometimes the swelling on one side of the face will disappear, only to be replaced by the opposite parotid gland becoming swollen. Whichever variation of symptoms occurs will make no difference to the immunity gained by an accurately diagnosed attack of mumps.

Eating or drinking can cause exquisite pain in the affected glands at the height of the infection.

A dry mouth is also a common complaint with an attack of mumps. This is due to the cessation of the normal amounts of saliva secreted by the affected salivary glands.

Investigations

Identification of the virus in the laboratory from saliva swabs gives positive proof of infection with the mumps virus. However, this is rarely done, as diagnosis can usually be made on clinical grounds.

Management

There is no specific treatment for an attack of mumps.

Analgesics are necessary to control the pain in cases where the parotid glands are swollen and tender. It is a good idea to give a painkiller about half an hour before a meal in order to reduce the pain caused by attempted salivary secretion from the inflamed gland. These useful drugs – such as paracetamol – will also help to lower fever, and so make the young patient feel more comfortable.

A **suitable diet** is also helpful during the height of an attack of mumps. **Fluids only** at the height of the swelling may be necessary. After this, **easily swallowed foods** such as soups, jellies, ice-cream and liquidized foods are helpful.

Children will need to **remain off school** until the worst of the swelling of the parotid glands has subsided. Infectivity is high until 4–5 days after the appearance of the swellings. After this time, schooling can be resumed with no risk to children in contact with the sufferer, always provided, of course, that the child is feeling completely well again.

Complications

Mumps has a poor record where complications are concerned. Indeed this is an important factor in an otherwise mild infectious disease.

Meningitis can be caused by the mumps virus. Occasionally, signs and symptoms of meningitis can be the first clue that a child is suffering from infection with the mumps virus. At other times, the meningitis occurs along with the swelling in the parotid glands or, again, after the worst of the swelling has subsided – as long as 10 days later. So this complication can be very variable in its onset. Signs of meningitis are **fever** (or a return of fever once the fever due to the original infection has subsided), **headache**, a **stiff neck** and, at times, a **sore throat**.

Hospital admission is usually necessary for a child with mumps meningitis. A lumbar puncture will confirm the diagnosis following laboratory examination of the cerebrospinal fluid thus obtained. As a side-effect, the lumbar puncture can bring rapid relief of headache.

Again, there is no specific treatment for mumps meningitis apart from good nursing care. (Antibiotics are of no value, as they are inactive against viral infections.) Recovery is usually complete but, sadly, occasional permanent brain damage can result from severe mumps meningitis.

Unilateral deafness can also be a residual handicap following mumps. Children who have had a severe attack of mumps and in whom deafness is suspected by the parents, or any child who has suffered from meningitis due to this infection, should receive a hearing test a few weeks following recovery from the infection. It can be all too easy to miss this complication, particularly in the younger age groups.

Orchitis is a further possible complication of an attack of mumps, but is rare before puberty. Here, one or both testes become acutely painful, red and swollen. Treatment is again non-specific. Support of the inflamed testes with appropriate firm bandages can be helpful, as can ice-bags applied to the hot swollen organ. Frequent painkillers can also be necessary. Sterility is by no means the inevitable outcome of mumps orchitis, as was once thought. Mothers of young boys should be firmly reassured on this point.

Pancreatitis, in which the pancreas becomes involved in the general infection, is a rare complication but can be the cause of acute abdominal pain during an attack of mumps. There is usually no permanent damage to this organ, but, very occasionally, diabetes can subsequently occur.

PREVENTION

Immunization against mumps is now possible with the **MMR** (measles, mumps and rubella) immunization. This is now a routine procedure in the UK at the age of around 1 year. Only one injection is necessary to ensure immunity. There is a risk of other members of the family acquiring any of the three infections from a younger, recently immunized, member.

Immunization should be postponed if the child due to receive the injection has any acute illness. Also, children receiving immunotherapy for other serious illnesses should not be given this immunization. The only other contraindication to receiving the vaccine is a proven allergy to the antibiotic neomycin or a serious reaction to eating eggs (egg products are used in the making of the vaccine). Mere dislike of eggs is no reason for omitting the vaccine!

The immunization can be given to children of any age.

The future

With the advent of immunization against mumps, this infection should eventually become an historical disease. In the USA, mumps vaccine has been given to children for over 20 years and there has been a dramatic drop in the number of infections and complications due to mumps reported. The most important factor must, of course, be the number of children suffering permanent consequences due to a severe complicated attack of mumps.

Nappy rash

Incidence

This is not a condition that has excited a good deal of research into the number of babies affected! But anyone having the care of babies will know that lucky is the infant who escapes nappy rash altogether.

Causation

There are a number of possibilities as to the cause of each particular type of nappy rash. By far the commonest, however, is the simple 'contact irritant' type. Other causative factors can be seborrhoeic dermatitis, added infection with *Candida* (thrush) and psoriasis.

Each will need a different treatment – see below.

Characteristics

'Contact irritant' nappy rash is the reaction of the relatively thin skin of the baby to constant contact with urine and faeces. Specific types of bacteria that are encouraged by the warm, damp atmosphere add to the irritation. These bacteria release ammonia, which is in itself a potent irritant. (A wet nappy often has the characteristic smell of ammonia.)

The rash is **red** and spreads over the **whole of the nappy area**, with characteristics **patches of clear skin** in the folds of the groin.

If terry-towelling nappies are being used these will need to be rinsed thoroughly after washing. Remnants of **washing powder** can also be an irritant cause of nappy rash.

Seborrhoeic dermatitis is a common cause of nappy rash. This can be readily confused with eczema. The most usual place for this to occur is on the scalp, where thick, yellowish crusts appear along the hair line. This is commonly know as 'cradle-cap'. Other areas affected are the creases of the body, such as behind the ears, around chubby necks, in elbow creases and also in the groin area. In this last – nappy – area, secondary infection with *Candida* is especially common.

Secondary infection with *Candida* ('thrush') – a yeast infection – can occur on top of an irritant type of nappy rash. The rash is then seen to have an added discrete red area with a well-defined edge. Newborn babies can be infected with thrush during delivery if the mother herself has a vaginal infection with this fungus. It is the baby's mouth under these circumstances that is most frequently affected, but spread to the nappy area can readily occur. With a *Candida* infection a cheesy-white substance can often be seen in the skin folds in addition to the red rash.

These three causes are by far the commonest reasons for nappy rash. On rare occasions a form of **psoriasis** can be seen in young babies in the nappy area. Characteristically, an existing mild nappy rash due to contact becomes more severe. Often, large, well-demarcated areas become bright red all over the nappy area, including the folds of the skin. It is usual under these circumstances for the typical lesions of psoriasis to appear elsewhere on the body.

MANAGEMENT

The mainstay of treatment of the common 'contact irritant' type of nappy rash is **frequent changing of the nappies.** This ensures that the skin is only in contact with urine and/or faeces for the minimum amount of time. Modern **disposable nappies** are preferable in this context to terry-towelling ones covered with plastic pants, which increase the tendency to a warm, moist environment highly favourable for the introduction of secondary infection. At each nappy change the baby's bottom needs to be **thoroughly cleaned and dried** and a **soothing cream,** such as one containing zinc, applied.

It is also helpful to allow the baby to **lie without a nappy** – in a warm room – for as long as possible each day.

A nappy rash due to **seborrhoeic dermatitis** will need the addition of a mild **hydrocortisone cream.** This will need also to be applied to other parts of the body affected. It is inadvisable to use this cream for extended periods of time on a number of different parts of the body. So if the nappy rash has not cleared within 1 week of this treatment, further advice as to the possible cause must be sought.

Added **infection with** *Candida* will need a different cream – **nystatin,** for example – to heal the rash. It is always a good idea, where thrush is giving rise to a nappy rash, to **check in the baby's mouth** to eliminate a possible infection also in that part of the body.

Psoriasis is a difficult skin condition to treat, and a number of preparations may need to be tried. This is, fortunately, a rare cause of nappy rash but one that needs to be remembered when a rash is proving difficult to treat by the usual means.

THE FUTURE

Nappy rash is a self-limiting condition and will no longer be a problem once nappies are discarded.

Otitis media

Alternative name

Middle ear infection.

Incidence

As with tonsillitis, for example, the true incidence of otitis media is not formally known. But any general practitioner will see a number of children every week with this condition.

Boys and girls of all races are equally affected.

The incidence of this infection is higher in cool, temperate climates during the winter months – when upper respiratory infections are at their height. Throat infections and/or tonsillitis frequently precede, or coexist with, acute otitis media.

History

Until routine treatment of otitis media with antibiotics from the 1950s onward, mastoiditis (infection in the bony mastoid process) was a relatively common condition. The mastoid process is situated behind and below the ears. This bony process readily becomes infected following a severe untreated otitis media. This infection was a serious side-effect of otitis media, with meningitis as a further possible sequel. Operation on the mastoid process was necessary to remove and drain the infected bone. Older people still show the scars of this procedure, along with the deafness that was often also the residual result.

Causation

The infecting organisms in otitis media can be either bacteria or viruses. Probably around half of the infections are due to a viral cause, but secondary bacterial infection is common.

Characteristics

Pain in the ear is the outstanding feature of acute otitis media. Even very young children accurately pinpoint the source of their pain as they clasp a hand over the affected ear, or rub it along the blanket or sheet. This pain can be one of the reasons for frequent waking in the night.

Fever, sometimes high, is also a frequent accompaniment of an acute ear infection.

Associated **coughs** and **colds** are again common. These are due to the easy spread of infection up the eustachian tube into the middle ear.

On examination with an auroscope in the early stages of the infection, the **eardrum** is seen to be **reddened** and covered with **dilated blood vessels**. Later, the delicate tissue of the drum will appear unusually **dull** and **congested** and bulge into the external auditory meatus. Ultimately, if no treatment has been available, the eardrum can **rupture** into the external auditory meatus. When this occurs, the pain will ease (because of the release of pressure) and a discharge of blood and pus will be seen flowing from the affected ear. Otitis media should never be allowed to reach this stage. Deafness can be a permanent late effect of rupture of the eardrum. The scar tissue that replaces the hole in the drum reduces the elasticity, and hence the adequate function, of this vital part of the hearing mechanism.

MANAGEMENT

Earache in children must always be regarded as an emergency, and medical help should be sought as soon as possible. Early treatment with **antibiotics** is essential if permanent damage to hearing is to be avoided. The pain from most attacks of otitis media usually clears up within 24 hours of starting treatment. But, in spite of this, it is important that the full course of a prescribed antibiotic should be finished, in order for the infection to be fully eradicated.

If the pain does not subside after a couple of days treatment with a specific antibiotic, it will be necessary to change to a different one – and so, once again, medical advice should be sought.

Analgesics such as paracetamol should be given in the early painful stages of otitis media. This will also help to reduce fever.

A **hearing test** should ideally be performed 3 months or so after a severe attack of otitis media. This is to ensure that the infection has not left the child with the complication of secretory otitis media.

COMPLICATIONS

Secretory otitis media ('glue ear')

Causation

The cause of secretory otitis media, as well as the possibility of this arising following an acute attack of otitis media, is unclear. It is thought that it is perhaps due to lack of proper drainage, via the eustachian tube, of secretions. This tiny tube can easily become blocked by mucus, or by swelling of the surrounding tissues, and so cause a build-up of sticky fluid in the middle ear. In turn, this fluid restricts the movement of the eardrum and so prevents sound-waves from travelling clearly to the nerves of hearing.

Characteristics

Secretory otitis media can be difficult to pinpoint. A child's hearing can be perfectly normal for several days, but for the next week or two can be very restricted due to a further build-up of fluid. The first signs of hearing loss can be **lack of attention** in school, or **turning up the sound** on the television to an unnecessarily high level. **Behaviour problems**, too, can have their basis in a hearing loss. The unfortunate child cannot hear clearly what is being said in class, becomes frustrated and so 'switches off' altogether or reacts in a generally antisocial manner. In younger children with this problem, the proper development of speech can be hindered.

Investigations

If secretory otitis media is suspected, an ear, nose and throat surgeon should see the child – to examine the eardrum and to perform specialized hearing tests such as impedance audiometry.

Management

This can be difficult, but includes trying the following.

- **Decongestant nose drops** and **antihistamine drugs** have both been prescribed over the years, but regretfully both can be less than satisfactory.
- In **myringotomy**, the eardrum is pierced, under a general anaesthetic, and the sticky fluid is withdrawn. Following this, a tiny ventilation tube or 'grommet' is placed in the eardrum to allow air into the cavity of the middle ear and so prevent the repeated build-up of fluid. Grommets rarely, if ever, need to be removed from their position in the eardrum. They fall out spontaneously, usually within a year to 18 months of their insertion. (They are so tiny that parents are usually quite unaware that they have been extruded. It is not until the ears are again examined with an auroscope that the grommets are found to be missing.)

  There has been much controversy over the years regarding the vexed question of whether or not children with grommets in their ears should be allowed to swim. It is unlikely that any harm will come to the middle ear if small amounts of water make their way into the external auditory canal – but much harm **can** come to a child if s/he cannot swim. It is wise, however, to ban such activities as diving under water if a child has grommets in his/her ears.
- **Hearing aids**, as a temporary measure, are gaining in popularity of recent years for the treatment of secretory otitis media (see Deafness, above).

THE FUTURE

Unless treatment for an acute attack of otitis media has been delayed or inadequate, or secretory otitis media has remained undiagnosed, most children will have normal hearing and few attacks of earache by the time they are 7 or 8 years of age.

PERTHES' DISEASE

ALTERNATIVE NAMES

Legg–Calvé–Perthes disease; coxa magna; osteochondritis.

INCIDENCE

Exact figures for this condition are not known, but it is thought that around 1 in every 2000 children is affected. Perthes' disease occurs in the 2–12 age group, but most cases are seen between the ages of 4 and 8 years. Boys are about four times more frequently affected than are girls. A few of the children with Perthes' disease have the condition in both hips.

While there is no discernible genetic cause, brothers and sisters of sufferers have a slightly higher chance of having the condition than does the general child population.

CAUSATION

Exactly why this condition should occur is uncertain. A temporary diminution in the blood-supply to the head of the femur, or thigh-bone, (the 'ball' of the 'ball-and-socket' hip joint) is the most probable cause. This, together with the compression exerted on this weight-bearing joint, are thought to be the two aetiological factors.

In addition to bony changes there is swelling of the surrounding soft tissues. These two factors eventually lead to destruction of the normal anatomy of the joint. It is these changes that give rise to the typical characteristics of the condition.

CHARACTERISTICS

Any child with a **limp** that lasts for longer than a few days should be investigated thoroughly. Obvious causes, e.g. a wound or a blister on the foot, can be easily eliminated. A limp, associated with an unusual, lurching gait, can be one of the first signs of Perthes' disease – even before the child complains of **pain**. This can be felt either in the affected joint itself or referred down the thigh into the knee.

This pain can vary in intensity from day to day, although it is usually consistently worse after exercise. (Strangely enough, the degree of pain seems to bear little relationship to the changes seen on X-ray. So it is important that even a mild degree of pain should be thoroughly investigated.)

On examination of the leg, there is found to be a **limitation of movement** of the hip. This is due to muscle spasm in an effort to protect the joint. The child will also actively dislike attempts to move the hip joint.

There is rarely any severe constitutional upset with Perthes' disease.

INVESTIGATIONS

X-ray of the affected joint will allow a definitive diagnosis, as the changes seen are quite typical of the condition. The space between the head of the thigh bone and the pelvis is seen to be wider than usual. This is due to the swelling of the surrounding soft tissues. With advanced disease, the usual smooth surface of the 'ball' of the hip joint is seen to be irregular and perhaps to contain cysts. It is when the actual growing part of the bone is affected that permanent damage – such as a shortening of the affected leg – can occur.

Following treatment, regular X-rays, at about 3-monthly intervals, are necessary to review progress. The hip joint will eventually heal and recalcify. The degree of residual disability will depend on the amount of bony destruction that has occurred during the active stages of the disease.

MANAGEMENT

In the initial stages of the disease, **bed-rest with the affected leg in traction** is necessary. The leg is held in an immobile raised position to allow the hip to heal without the stresses and strains on the joint that inevitably occur when the child is walking or running. **Physiotherapy** is vital during this stage to ensure that the muscles in the legs do not become weak during this period of inactivity.

Analgesics of appropriate type and dosage depending on the child's age and weight should be given if pain is severe.

Schooling for children of school age with Perthes' disease will need to be kept up to date because of the unavoidable absences from school during treatment. Contact with the child's school can often be arranged, with appropriate work and activities sent to the child. This will obviate much of the boredom and frustration of enforced inactivity as well as keeping the young patient in touch with events at school.

Depending on the stage of the disease as seen on X-ray, the hip can eventually be immobilized in a special type of **splint** with the leg held outwards and rotated inwards. This is an incredibly awkward position, but it is surprising how quickly children adapt to it and how mobile they become! With some rearrangement in the classroom and a sympathetic teacher, the child can once again attend school. This form of immobilization will need to be continued for several months.

Time off from school will be necessary for continuing **physiotherapy** to ensure that unused muscles do not become weak. Again, sympathetic understanding on the part of the child's teacher is vital.

Emotional support of both parents and child will be necessary during this long period of immobilization of the affected leg. Encouragement, from orthopaedic consultant, general practitioner, health visitor and school can do much to help.

The future

Depending on the severity of the Perthes' disease there may be, in a few children, some **shortening** of the leg on the affected side. This will only occur if the actual growing part of the bone has been affected. Usually, little effect is noticed even if this has occurred.

In later adult life, following Perthes' disease in childhood, **osteoarthritis** in the affected hip may occur earlier than is usual.

Related conditions

Osteochondritis is not confined to the hip joint. Other joints, and particular parts of bones, can also be affected. The disease process is exactly the same as in Perthes' disease. These osteochondrites are given different names according to the bone affected.

Osgood–Schlatter's disease

This is osteochondritis of the tibial tubercle – the small bony projection in the shin bone just below the knee.

Osgood-Schlatter's disease usually occurs in boys around the time of puberty. There is a painful swelling in this position on the leg, causing the boy to walk with a limp. X-ray changes are similar to those seen in Perthes' disease.

Treatment is by immobilization in plaster for 6–8 weeks, or temporary restriction of vigorous activity in mild cases. Following this, a gradual return to full activity, over the succeeding 2 months or so, is advisable. The help of a physiotherapist is valuable in strengthening muscles weakened by inactivity.

Sever's disease

This time it is the heel bone that is involved. Again, X-ray changes are similar, and the child will find walking painful. Once again, this condition occurs more commonly in adolescence. A walking plaster may be necessary for around 6 weeks to relieve pain, although fitting a raised heel to the shoe can sometimes give sufficient relief.

Kohler's disease

A small bone in the foot is the site of the osteochondritis in Kohler's disease. Boys between the ages of 3 and 8 years are most commonly affected. Again, a limp, with local pain and tenderness in the foot, are the symptoms of Kohler's disease. Walking tends to aggravate the pain.

A 6–8 week period of immobilization in a walking plaster will promote recovery.

The future

All the above conditions heal readily and leave no permanent after-effects.

SELF-HELP GROUP

Perthes' Association
15 Recreation Road
Guildford, GU1 1HE
Tel. 01483 306 637
Fax 01483 508 213.

Pityriasis

Incidence

Pityriasis rosea (pityriasis alba is a similar condition, but is rarely seen) is an uncommon condition, but can give rise to much concern because of the extensive rash that is the main feature of the disease. Older children – over the age of 10 years – are the most usual sufferers. Pityriasis is frequently found during adolescence.

All races are equally affected, as are both sexes. Some authorities say that one attack of pityriasis confers immunity for life, but this is by no means necessarily so.

History

Pityriasis has been recognized for centuries. Pityriasis is a word derived from the Greek meaning 'bran'. This aptly describes the flaky scales on the skin characteristic of the condition.

Causation

Strangely enough, the exact cause of pityriasis is not clearly known. Various ideas have had their vogue, and range from a fungal infection through an allergic manifestation to a viral origin. It is now thought that this last is the true cause, although no specific virus has so far been isolated.

Cases of pityriasis tend to occur in clusters. This adds extra force to the infective theory.

Characteristics

Characteristically, pityriasis begins with one lesion on the skin, known as the **herald patch**. This is a single, round eruption occurring anywhere on the body, but most usually on the chest, back or upper limbs. This patch can be anything up to 10 cm in diameter, and has a typical scaly appearance, often with a patch of clear skin in the centre. (If seen alone, this can easily be confused with a patch of discoid eczema.)

Within a week or two an **extensive rash** develops all over the body. Fortunately, hands, feet and face are usually spared, although the rash does occasionally extend to these exposed sites of the body. More of the rash tends to appear every 2 or 3 days for around a week. This rapidity of spread can be quite alarming, particularly in the skin-conscious adolescent. The rash **may be irritant**, but this is not always the case.

The rash will gradually disappear, but it will be between 3 and 8 weeks before the skin is finally completely clear – again a source of much distress. As with the herald patch, the lesions will clear initially in the centres, leaving a ruff of bran-like scales around the edges of the spots. Eventually the rash will disappear completely, leaving no residual trace of the once extensive eruption.

Very occasionally, there may be a mild fever and a general feeling of ill-health before the rash becomes apparent, but this is unusual.

MANAGEMENT

There is little that can be done to speed the cure of this trivial, but nevertheless distressing, condition. If irritation is a problem, a **steroid cream** can be helpful, or an **antihistamine** given at night.

Reassurance that, within a few weeks, the rash will completely disappear is important. As mentioned previously, recurrence is rare, but can occur – often many years later.

There is no need for children with pityriasis to stay away from **school**, although it is important that teachers – and other parents! – are reassured that the extensive rash is not infectious.

THE FUTURE

There are no adverse effects following an attack of pityriasis rosea.

PSORIASIS

INCIDENCE

Psoriasis is known worldwide and affects people of all races. It is usually thought of as a disease of adult life but can, in fact, occur in the youngest of children. In babies a particular type of nappy rash, which is very resistant to the usual forms of treatment, is thought to be often due to psoriasis.

Both sexes can be affected; girls more often than boys. There is often a strong family history of the condition.

HISTORY

It is possible that some of the leprous lesions described in antiquity may have been due to psoriasis.

CAUSATION

Psoriasis is considered to be a dominantly inherited disorder. If one parent has the condition, one out of four of their children will stand a chance of inheriting the disease. (Regretfully there is no way of predicting which child will be affected. Similarly if, for example, the first child in the family has psoriasis, this does not mean that the next three children will be free of the condition. The chances are 1 in 4 for each successive child.)

Faults in immunological function and also hormonal imbalance are thought to be implicated in psoriasis.

The onset of psoriasis frequently occurs following a bout of infection or any other form of stress, e.g. an accident or a bereavement.

CHARACTERISTICS

In children, psoriasis usually begins in a slightly different form from the lesions seen in the adult form of the disease. The **rash** consists of small patches, or 'drops' (the name **guttate psoriasis** – *gutta* meaning 'a drop' in Latin – is applied to these early lesions). They can occur anywhere on the body, including the face.

As the child matures, the rash changes its characteristics to the more adult form. This consists of larger **plaques** with a **white, scaly surface**, mainly on the knees, elbows and scalp. In children, the rash of psoriasis is often preceded by an **upper respiratory tract infection** with the streptococcus bacteria.

When psoriasis affects armpits, groins or the napkin area in babies, the scaliness is less evident and the rash is red and angry-looking. Typically, the edges of the rash of psoriasis have a well-defined margin. The rash does not itch.

Psoriasis is a condition that fluctuates in severity throughout life. Periods of stress or infection will often increase the amount of rash seen. Psoriasis is **not an infectious condition,** and this should be explained fully to parents and teachers as well as to the children themselves.

MANAGEMENT

Psoriasis is a skin condition for which there is no complete cure. But much improvement can be gained by the various forms of treatment available. It is important that both child and parent should understand this so that the disappointment is not too great when the rash recurs. **Encouragement** to persevere with treatment and **emotional support** are vital as the child matures and learns to live with the inherited skin condition.

Sunlight usually has a beneficial effect on psoriasis. So children and adolescents should be encouraged to expose arms and legs with a psoriasis rash in summer time rather than covering up the scaly lesions in an attempt to hide them from their contemporaries.

Preparations in the form of ointments or pastes – based on tar and salicylic acid – are the most suitable for use in children. There are a wide range of these preparations and trial will decide which one is of the most benefit to each individual child.

Weak **steroid preparations** are also useful. These should be used for a short time only, because of the possible side-effects that can occur with these drugs. Unfortunately, there is often a relapse once these preparations are withdrawn.

If the child has an upper respiratory tract infection at a time when the rash is at its worst, a course of **penicillin** will often clear the rash as well as curing the respiratory tract infection.

Long-term follow-up of children with this unpleasant condition is important, preferably by the same doctor, who will be able to reassure and encourage, knowing the previous condition of the child's skin.

Children with psoriasis can suffer from taunts at **school.** This will require sympathetic handling by teachers, who should be informed of the non-infectious – and recurrent – nature of the condition.

Certain **careers** will be inadvisable for children with psoriasis. They should be advised against considering careers in chemistry, in the beauty industry or in certain artistic activities when the time comes for choices to be made.

COMPLICATIONS

Psoriasis is regretfully a lifelong condition that is characterized by periods of remission and relapse. Treatment will need to be varied according to the position and severity of the lesions at any one time.

Arthritis can be a long-term complication of psoriasis.

The Psoriasis Association
7 Milton Street
Northampton, NN2 7JG
Tel. 01604 711129.

PYLORIC STENOSIS

ALTERNATIVE NAME

Congenital hypertrophic pyloric stenosis. (This alternative name is unsuitable, because the word 'congenital' implies a condition present at birth, whereas the symptoms of pyloric stenosis only very rarely begin before 2 or 3 weeks of age. Also, the condition has never been reported in a stillborn baby.)

INCIDENCE

The incidence of pyloric stenosis is four times as high in boys as in girls. It is thought that about 1 in every 250 male babies are affected, with a figure of 1 in 1000 in girls.

Pyloric stenosis is most commonly found in Caucasian races and is rare in Asiatic peoples. In Chinese babies, for example, the condition is virtually unknown.

Surgery for pyloric stenosis is one of the commonest abdominal operations to be performed in the early weeks of life.

CAUSATION

While no direct genetic link has been found, there appears to be definite family factors at work. It is probable that a number of genes are involved and also that there is some sex linkage – this latter showing up as the higher incidence in boys.

HISTORY

Until surgery became possible to relieve – and cure – pyloric stenosis, many babies succumbed. The obstruction to the passage of food into the intestine meant that starvation, dehydration and severe electrolytic upset were the result.

The results of Ramstedt's operation for pyloric stenosis were first published in 1912, and soon after this the operation became routine procedure.

CHARACTERISTICS

The pylorus is that part of the stomach leading into the duodenum (the first part of the small intestine). It consists of a thick band of muscular tissue, which opens periodically to allow the contents of the stomach (where the initial processes of digestion take place) through into the small intestine, where further digestion and absorption takes place.

Hypertrophy (enlargement) of this muscular band effectively narrows the lumen of this canal, so that emptying of the stomach is initially delayed and eventually ceases altogether. These facts lead to the symptoms.

- **Projectile vomiting** starts at around 2–3 weeks of age. The vomiting is violent and can be projected several feet. Immediately after vomiting the baby will be anxious to feed again. This is in direct contradistinction to vomiting due to an infective process.
- As the condition progresses **weight loss** occurs and general **failure to thrive.**
- **Constipation** due to lack of any nutrients passing through into the intestine becomes evident within a few days. The baby with pyloric stenosis has a typical hungry, worried expression – hardly surprising when the basic necessities of life are missing!
- Diagnosis can be confirmed by observing a **swelling**, which can be both seen and felt, passing across the top of the baby's abdomen as a feed is given.

X-ray studies used to be done to confirm the diagnosis, but today **ultrasound** is the diagnostic method used.

MANAGEMENT

Ramstedt's operation, performed under general anaesthesia, is safe and has excellent results. In this procedure the enlarged muscle of the pylorus is divided, allowing fluids to pass through uninterrupted. Babies will be able to feed normally within 3–4 hours following the operation, and are usually allowed home after 24–36 hours. Postoperatively, feeding is best done with the baby in a sitting position, and leaning towards the right. This will assist in the emptying of the stomach.

Previous to Ramstedt's operation, antispasmodic drugs were used, with generally unsatisfactory results. They have no place in modern treatment.

COMPLICATIONS

If the vomiting has been severe and prolonged before operation, **irritation of the stomach lining** can occur. This can, at times, cause post-operative vomiting. Stomach wash-outs usually cure this problem.

THE FUTURE

There are no known after-effects in later life due to pyloric stenosis in infancy, although some authorities have suggested that the incidence of peptic ulcer is higher.

Rashes

Incidence

No overall incidence can be quoted, as there are a multitude of different causes for a rash. Probably every single child has had some kind of rash at some time during childhood.

Causation

The causes of skin rashes can be divided into two broad categories. Some rashes are associated with, and part of the signs of, a wider illness. The infectious fevers of childhood are good examples of this. Then there are all the rashes that arise in the skin itself with only little, if any, involvement of the rest of the body.

Rashes differ in their appearance according to the cause. There are five different types of rash:

- **macules,** which are flat lesions that have a pink or red colour and cannot be individually felt;
- **papules,** which are round, raised and red and so can be easily felt when running a hand over the surface of the skin;

(These two types of rash often appear together.)

- **vesicles,** which are round, raised and filled with fluid; this in turn can be clear, or opaque because of pus formation;
- **petechiae,** which are spots rather like small bruises and do not whiten when pressed with a finger – larger areas of this type of rash are termed **purpura;**
- other, more **specific rashes** as seen in eczema or fungal conditions.

Each condition having a rash as part of the disease will have one or other of these types of rash.

Characteristics

Rashes associated with a wider illness

The following infections all have a **maculopapular** rash (a mixture of macules and papules) as part of the features of the condition:

- measles, rubella, scarlet fever, fifth disease, roseola infantum, Kawasaki disease.

The rash in each of these illnesses is distinctive in position on the body and timing, and is also associated with other symptoms specific to the individual condition. Some viral infections that have no specific symptoms other than general debility, loss of appetite with maybe a cough and a runny nose can also have this type of associated rash. This disappears as the infections clears.

Conditions that have a rash consisting of **vesicles** are:

- chickenpox, some allergic conditions.

Petechiae is the rash most seriously associated with meningococcal meningitis. Henoch–Schönlein purpura also has this type of rash – as the name implies.

All these conditions are described individually in other parts of this text.

Rashes associated only with the skin

There may be a mild constitutional upset with these conditions, but usually it is only the skin that is affected.

Impetigo and **molluscum contagiosum** both have macules or papules as the specific rash. Impetigo is discussed elsewhere (see above). Molluscum contagiosum is a rash most commonly seen in the 2–5-year age group, and is due to a pox-type viral infection. The rash is discrete, round and pearly white in colour. It most usually arises in the armpit area and down the sides of the chest. This infection is transmitted from child to child in swimming baths or by siblings sharing a warm bath at bedtime. The child is not at all unwell and this rash will eventually clear spontaneously. Showering instead of bathing and the temporary avoidance of swimming baths will prevent reinfection and prolongation of the rash.

Eczema, pityriasis and **psoriasis** all have a very specific type of rash, and all tend to have a very scaly surface. These again are described elsewhere in the text.

Ringworm and **thrush** are two relatively common skin rashes that are both caused by a fungus. Ringworm is – as the name suggests – a circle of small bright-red papules surrounding a white centre. This infection can be picked up from pets such as dogs, cats and hamsters, as well as cattle – and other children. There is no added constitutional upset with ringworm, but treatment with antifungal creams is necessary to prevent spread – both in the individual and also spread to other children (and adults). Thrush is a common fungal infection often found in young babies in the mouth or the nappy area. Further information can be found above under Nappy rash.

There is one further unusual skin infection, which is caused by a specific bacteria of the staphylococcal strain. This is known as **staphylococcal scalded skin syndrome (SSS)** because of the striking resemblance to skin that has been scalded by hot liquid. The appearance of the skin in this condition is quite unlike any other condition with a skin rash. Fortunately, only the superficial layer of the skin is involved, so fluid loss – a dangerous side-effect of a severe scald – is not a problem. The child will, however, be in a good deal of pain with this infection and will also be running a fever. Within a week the top layer of skin will peel off, leaving normal skin that has no visible scarring as a result. Penicillin is needed to treat this condition and powerful painkillers are usually needed in the initial acutely painful stage.

Rashes in children are notoriously difficult to diagnose, but the associated symptoms can make the picture clear within a few hours or days. Enquiries into similar symptoms in other members of the family will often be a help with rashes due to infectious disease.

Roseola infantum

ALTERNATIVE NAMES

Sixth disease; three-day fever; exanthum subitum.

INCIDENCE

The exact incidence of roseola infantum is not known. It probably occurs more frequently than is thought, as the symptoms can be easily confused with a number of other conditions that are also associated with a rash. It is a disease of infancy – as the most commonly used name implies.

CAUSATION

Roseola infantum is caused by a virus – the Human herpes virus 6. It is possible to confirm the diagnosis by cultivation of the virus from the blood of affected children. This is rarely done, however, as the disease runs a brief course with only very few instances of complications. Diagnosis is made clinically by the characteristic symptoms.

CHARACTERISTICS

The infection begins suddenly with a relatively **high fever** – between 38.9°C and 40.6°C. Associated with this, the child will be **off food** and generally **unwell** and **irritable**, especially when the fever is at its height.

This fever last for 3–5 days and then falls suddenly back to normal. As the fever drops a **rash** appears. This is a discrete red rash that occurs mainly on the **torso and neck**, although occasionally the arms, legs and face are also involved. In direct contrast to measles, there are **no signs inside the child's mouth** of a specific rash, although there may be ulcers on the tongue and soft palate. Also, again unlike measles, the rash does not coalesce but remains as **discrete markings** on the skin.

In addition to these signs the lymph **glands at the back of the neck** are often enlarged. This can make the differential diagnosis from rubella difficult – and indeed the two conditions are frequently confused. The age of the child and the sudden onset of high fever before the rash appears, however, should make the difference clear.

INVESTIGATIONS

An uncomplicated attack of roseola infantum usually requires no further investigation, the diagnosis being made from the signs and symptoms. If blood is taken, this will show a rise in the white blood cell count during the days when a fever is present. Viral studies can be done, but this is not a routine procedure.

MANAGEMENT

There is no specific treatment for roseola infantum. The main risk is that of a **febrile convulsion** occurring, due to the sudden rise in temperature. If this does occur, attempts need to be made to **cool the child** by removing all excess clothing, avoiding hot, stuffy rooms and sponging down with tepid water. If a convulsion does occur this should be reported to the child's doctor, who may prescribe a **sedative** to be given rectally if necessary and/or if the convulsion recurs.

Apart from the treatment of this complication, a **light diet** with **plenty of fluids** and an appropriate drug to help lower the temperature – such as **paracetamol** – is all that needs to be done.

COMPLICATIONS

These are rare, the main one being a febrile convulsion, as described above. Very rarely **encephalitis** (when the infection affects the brain) can occur. Here, the child will not make the usual quick recovery, but will become progressively more ill, with further convulsions being a feature. Medical aid under these circumstances is urgently needed.

PREVENTION

There is no vaccine available for roseola infantum. This would seem unnecessary for such a comparatively benign disease with few serious complications or side-effects.

THE FUTURE

There are no long-term sequelae due to roseola infantum. apart from the extremely rare effects of encephalitis.

Rubella

Alternative name

German measles.

Incidence

The true incidence of rubella is exceedingly difficult to determine as many of these infections are so mild as to pass unnoticed. From studies on antibody levels to the infection in adult populations, it is thought that around 90% of town-dwellers have suffered from an attack of rubella in their youth – many of them probably without realizing this. People who live in more rural areas have a lower incidence because of their decreased likelihood of meeting the infection.

It is probable that rubella is primarily a disease of childhood, the infection most probably being acquired between the ages of 5 and 12 years – the primary school years. Rubella has been a notifiable disease since 1988.

History

Rubella has been known for many years. The rather unfortunate name of 'German measles' came about through the early descriptions of the infection in Germany, and by a slight, superficial resemblance to measles. In fact, the infection is no more common in Germany than anywhere else, and certainly has no relationship at all to measles! It was only in 1962 that the rubella virus was finally identified and cultured – surprisingly late for so common a disease.

The importance of this mild disease is the devastating effects it can have on the unborn baby if the mother contracts the infection during the first 3 months of pregnancy. These effects were discovered, through brilliant detective work, by an Australian doctor in the 1960s.

Causation

Rubella is caused by a virus. The incubation period of the infection is between 14 and 21 days.

Characteristics

The typical **rash** is often the first sign of the disease in children. This begins on the face, and rapidly spreads over the chest, back and, to a lesser extent, the limbs. The rash is fine and pink, with the spots in some cases becoming so extensive that they coalesce. The length of time that the rash persists is very variable. It is usually apparent for anything up to 5 days, but can occasionally be so transient as to not be seen at all or to last merely a few hours.

Swelling of the lymph **glands in the neck** is a constant feature of infection with the rubella virus. This enlargement can precede the appearance of the rash. These swollen glands can be tender, particularly the ones at the back of the neck. In fact, tenderness on combing a child's hair is often the first clue that a rubella infection is present.

Mild fever, headache and general **malaise** can accompany the infection, but frequently the child may not feel any ill effects of the disease.

Management

There is no specific treatment for an attack of rubella and, indeed, this is rarely required because of the mild nature of the disease.

Analgesics may be necessary for headache and fever control – in appropriate dosage and type for the individual child. (Do remember that aspirin compounds should not be used for children under the age of 12 years, because of the possibility of Reye's syndrome.)

Children should be **kept away from school** during the acute stage of the disease when the rash is in evidence or they are feeling unwell. With a fleeting rash and a mild infection this can be difficult to implement. But if there is any suggestion that a child may have rubella the **school should be informed**. Any pregnant teacher can then take steps to determine her immunity – or otherwise – to rubella, if this has not already been done.

Complications

Rubella has a very low complication rate. A transient **arthritis** can occur in the small joints of the body – hands, wrists and ankles in particular. This occurs more frequently with adults suffering from the disease, but can also occur in children.

Encephalitis (inflammation of the brain) can occur following rubella, but is very rare.

Epistaxis (nose bleeding), **haematuria** (blood in the urine) or **purpura** (small bleeding spots under the skin) can also occur in association with an attack of rubella, due to changes in the blood from the infection. This will resolve without specific treatment.

Prevention

Rubella is a disease that is preventable by **immunization**. It is important that the highest levels of protection by immunization are reached in order to reduce to a minimum the number of babies born with the 'rubella syndrome'. This is a devastating condition in which babies can be born deaf, blind and/or with a heart condition if their mothers have contracted rubella during the first 3 months of pregnancy. By ensuring that the pool of infection among young children is reduced, there is less likelihood of rubella being a possibility at this time in a normal reproductive life.

Until 1988, all schoolgirls in the UK were offered immunization against rubella at 10–14 years of age in order to protect them during the critical child-bearing years. Since this date, however, immunization against rubella has been given as part of the **MMR** (measles, mumps and rubella) injection between the ages of 1 and 2 years with a booster at 4 to 5 years of age. Rubella immunization is still available to girls between 10 and 14 years of age and also to those women who on blood testing are found to be non-immune to rubella, for the foreseeable future. This will continue until the 'catch-up' time when all babies have had this immunization routinely.

THE FUTURE

There are virtually no long-term effects following an attack of rubella, apart from the possible effects on the newborn baby if rubella is contracted during pregnancy. It is to be hoped that a time can be visualized when no further rubella syndrome babies are born, as a result of the elimination of this particular infection.

Scabies

Incidence

Scabies is an infestation with a mite. It occurs worldwide and is especially common in the developing world and in places where hygiene is less than perfect.

Scabies is unusual in that there appears to be wide fluctuations in incidence. Epidemics seem to arise about every 15 years or so. In recent years the incidence of scabies has markedly increased. These facts are possibly due to a form of natural immunity to the mite that develops among communities. The recent higher reported incidence indicates that this immunity may be on the decline.

January, April and November, for some obscure reason, are the months in the UK when most cases occur.

History

Scabies has been known since the 17th century. It is said to be the first disease in man for which the cause was known – i.e. infestation with the mite *Sarcoptes scabiei*.

Causation

Infestation with a specific mite is the cause of the symptoms. The adult female scabies mite is only around 0.5 mm long and has been graphically described as closely resembling a minute tortoise. This female burrows into the skin by initially standing on her head to gain entry into the skin and then burrowing along parallel to the surface of the skin. As she travels along, eggs are laid. These burrowing activities leave S-shaped tracks, which are visible to the naked eye and are typical of the condition. It can be difficult to see the tracks as they are so small and are also frequently overlaid with skin inflammation due to scratching.

Characteristics

Scabies is characterized by intense **itching**. This is worst at night when the body is warm. The irritation not only occurs in the positions where the mite is active, but can occur all over the body. This is thought to be due to a generalized hypersensitivity to the presence of the mite.

The **rash** associated with scabies is very variable. For example, raised blistery spots can be seen alongside raised red discrete spots, all overlaid with scratch marks caused by an attempt to quell the overwhelming irritation. Also, as a result of this scratching, the skin can become infected. With all these various lesions on the skin it can often be very difficult to find the 'burrows' of the scabies mite that is the basic cause of all the problems.

The **most usual sites** for scabies to occur are around the insides of the wrists, under the arms, between the fingers and around those areas of the body where clothes fit tightly – such as waist and groin. Other areas of the body can also show signs of the infestation, but usually the palms of the hands, the soles of the feet and the face and scalp regions remain clear. (One exception to this latter fact is when the infestation occurs in young babies. In these infants, the face and hands are often also affected.)

The diagnosis of scabies is often delayed because of the difficulty of finding the typical burrows of the scabies mite among all the possible differing lesions on the skin. The marked irritation should arouse suspicion, and especially if more than one member of the family – or nursery/school class – is having this problem. The infestation is passed on from person to person by close physical contact. Scabies cannot be 'caught' from clothing or bedding.

MANAGEMENT

There are a number of preparations available with which to treat scabies. Benzyl benzoate emulsion is probably the best known and most effective. This emulsion should be applied to the whole of the child's body with the exception of the head and neck. It should be applied following a warm bath and allowed to dry on the body. Treatment should be given on two consecutive nights to ensure that all the mites – in all stages of development – are eradicated. If there is a good deal of secondary infection as a result of frequent and persistent scratching – which can be almost impossible to control – an appropriate **antibiotic** will need to be prescribed. The **whole family** may need to be treated if there is any suggestion that they too are affected by the presence of a rash and persistent irritation. Nightwear and bedlinen will need to be laundered in the usual way following treatment with benzyl benzoate in order to remove the unpleasant odour.

An unfortunate manifestation of scabies is that, even though adequate treatment has been carried out, the itch may still persist for several weeks. A specific cream is available that will help to control this unpleasant aspect of the condition.

Schooling can continue as usual once the treatment has been undertaken.

Scarlet fever

Incidence

The exact incidence of scarlet fever is not known, but the infection is certainly far less in evidence than 50 years ago. At this time, scarlet fever was a much-dreaded disease, both from the point of view of the severity of the illness and for the possible complications – rheumatic fever and glomerulonephritis. These complications were frequently seen because of the absence of any specific treatment for scarlet fever.

Also, over the years the virulence of the bacteria causing this infection appears to have diminished, again making the disease less serious when it does occur.

Scarlet fever is an uncommon condition in the preschool child.

History

Between the two world wars, fever, or isolation, hospitals were an integral part of the health scene. Patients, both children and adults, were nursed in these isolation units in an attempt to control the spread of the infections. Before the advent of antibiotics, isolation of the sufferers had a large part to play in the control of infectious disease. Scarlet fever patients formed a large part of the inmates of these fever hospitals. Today, antibiotic treatment has replaced the need for such isolation facilities.

Causation

Scarlet fever is caused by a particular strain of the group A beta-haemolytic *Streptococcus* bacterium. (Beta-haemolytic streptococci are classified according to the changes seen when the bacteria are grown under laboratory conditions.) These bacteria are also among the organisms that cause the skin infection impetigo.

The bacteria are usually passed on from child to child by droplet infection. They can also be passed on via a wound, burn or skin infection contaminated with the particular bacteria. The incubation period is a short one; 1–7 days is quoted, but 3–4 days is the more usual time at which symptoms appear after contact with a sufferer.

Characteristics

Scarlet fever usually starts very abruptly with the sudden onset of:

- headache;
- very sore throat;

- **fever**, which can be very high for the first few days of the illness;
- **vomiting**.

These features can also be seen at the onset of any severe throat infection or tonsillitis. It is when the typical **rash** of scarlet fever appears that a definite diagnosis can be made. This is usually on the second day of the illness. The rash is typically one of a generalized redness (or erythema) of the skin with specific small spots of an intense scarlet colour (hence the name of this condition.) The rash begins on the face and rapidly spreads to the neck and chest and then on to the limbs. Armpits, elbow creases and groin all show a dense concentration of the rash. Also, the rash on the face is quite typical in as much as the area around the mouth is free of the bright red rash.

The rash starts to fade after 2 or 3 days. Following this, in severe cases, the skin where the rash has been at its height begins to peel off, leaving clear skin underneath. Mild attacks do not show this desquamation process. (In olden days this peeled skin was much feared, as it was thought to carry the infection. It is now recognized that the shed skin is sterile.). With the disappearance of the rash the young patient will begin to feel better. The fever will drop, sore throat and headache will disappear and appetite will improve. The **tonsils** and whole throat will be reddened, with white patches covering the surface. **Ears** can also be affected along with the generalized throat infection, and are seen to be reddened on examination.

The appearance of the **tongue** is quite unique in scarlet fever. Initially it is coated with a white, fur-like substance with the bright red spots of the infection showing through. At this stage it is termed the 'white strawberry' tongue! In a couple of days the whole tongue becomes red – the 'red strawberry' tongue.

INVESTIGATIONS

Throat swabs can be taken and sent to the laboratory for the infection organism to be determined if the diagnosis is uncertain. But this is rarely done as scarlet fever can so readily be diagnosed from the clinical signs and symptoms.

MANAGEMENT

Antibiotic treatment has transformed scarlet fever from a serious disease, with the possibility of long-term complications, to a relatively mild, although unpleasant, illness. Penicillin is the antibiotic usually prescribed to treat this infection, but erythromycin can also be used for children who are allergic to penicillin.

Within 48 hours of starting treatment, there is no longer any possibility of passing on the infection to another member of the family.

It is important that the antibiotic treatment is continued for 10 days in order to completely eradicate the bacteria. There is no need to give penicillin as a prophylactic measure to other children in the family, unless they are taking steroids for some other condition. Under these circumstances they should be given penicillin to ensure that they do not suffer an attack from the *Streptococcus* bacillus.

Analgesics – usually in the form of some paracetamol compound for children – can be given to relieve headache and sore throat. This drug will also help to lower the temperature, and so will make the young patient feel more comfortable.

A **light diet** with **plenty of cool fluids** is helpful during the stage of the acute sore throat. The child will usually have little, or no, appetite for solid food, but it is important that adequate fluids should be given to prevent dehydration, which can occur, especially if the fever is high.

Bed-rest for the first 2 or 3 days, when the temperature is at its height, will probably be the most comfortable place for the child. As soon as wishes to get up are expressed, quiet play in a warm room is quite satisfactory.

Schooling can be resumed as soon as the child's general health and energy have returned to normal. This includes, of course, the complete disappearance of the rash, no further sore throat and a return to normal appetite and interest in usual activities.

COMPLICATIONS

With immediate and adequate treatment with penicillin, or other appropriate drug, these are uncommon.

Acute otitis media, in which there is earache and redness on examination of the eardrum, can occur as part of the initial symptomatology. The penicillin will rapidly cure this possible complication.

Sinusitis and/or **enlarged neck glands** can also occur following scarlet fever.

In the preantibiotic era, **glomerulonephritis** often occurred a few weeks or months following the primary illness. In this condition, the kidneys can be seriously damaged and leave the sufferer with long-term problems. This rarely, if ever, happens today. Similarly, **rheumatic fever**, which frequently affected the heart, was a feared complication of scarlet fever. Again, this is virtually unknown today. **Bronchopneumonia** was again a common complication. But antibiotics ensure that this rarely happens nowadays.

PREVENTION

There is no immunization available against scarlet fever. The causative organism, *Streptococcus* bacteria, are to be found in 10–20% of the throats of perfectly fit children. With such a widespread finding, immunization would be difficult. And as the treatment is so relatively easy and successful, there would not seem to be the need for a vaccine. Early diagnosis and treatment is the mainstay to prevent the serious complications of the disease.

The Future

An attack of scarlet fever, as discussed above, rarely leads to any long-term complications these days. One attack does not necessarily lead to immunity from acquiring a sore throat with *Streptococcus* as the causative organism, but the full-blown picture of scarlet fever rarely occurs more than once.

SLEEP DISTURBANCE

INCIDENCE

Problems with night-time waking and difficulty in getting a child off to sleep at bedtime are extremely common. Recent research has indicated that up to 20% of 2-year-olds wake in the night at least five times every week. Both boys and girls seem to be equally affected.

Subjectively, it would seem that only a very few fortunate parents have no problem at all with the sleeping patterns of their children.

CAUSATION

Illness of any kind, even the common head cold, will give rise to sleeping difficulties – as for anyone of whatever age. A stuffy nose and an irritating cough are not conducive to quiet sleep, and a fever will make anyone restless.

The **temperament of the child** also has a bearing on sleep patterns. The overactive child will have as much difficulty in getting off to sleep as in controlling overactive behaviour during the day. At the other end of the scale, quiet children may be those for whom the 'worries' of the day prevent sleep.

Anxiety in parents regarding sleep can also adversely affect the child's ability to settle satisfactorily at night. Parents who frequently 'pop in' to the child throughout the evening will only aggravate the feelings of insecurity that may be affecting the child regarding sleep. Worrying events during the previous day can also play on a child's mind and prevent sleep. This can happen if, for example, a much loved grandparent has recently died. The child can feel frightened to go to sleep under these circumstances in case they, too, may die.

CHARACTERISTICS

Sleep problems fall into two main groups:

- difficulty in getting to sleep;
- frequent waking during the night.

Both these aspects can give rise to much parental concern. In the former, they seem to have no time at all to themselves after a hard day if their child will not settle to sleep at a reasonable time. Frequent waking, too, can lead to complete parental exhaustion if this continues for months on end. The child can make up for lost sleep during the day, but not so for the poor exhausted parents.

Other sleep problems include the following.

- **Nightmares**. These are unpleasant dreams that wake the child – and the rest of the household! – screaming in fright. The dream will be vividly remembered and much reassurance is needed to calm the child and induce sleep again.
- **Night terrors** are quite different from nightmares. Here the child will awake terrified, but does not respond when spoken to and at times seems even not to see parents. This altered state of consciousness can last for up to 10 minutes, with the child being quite unable to be comforted. Eventually sleep will return and the child will wake in the morning with no recollection of the night's events or the distress that was so obviously felt at the time. Night terrors most frequently affect children between the ages of 4 and 7 years.
- **Sleep walking** is a further sleep disturbance that usually affects older children – from around 8 years upwards into the teen years. The child gets up from bed with a fixed, blank expression, does not respond to anyone and walks downstairs or into another room for no apparent reason. It is difficult to waken the child under these conditions and this should not be attempted (see below). Eventually the sleep walker will return to bed and – once again – be quite unaware the following morning of the events of the night.

MANAGEMENT

Difficulty in getting to sleep can be helped by a **calm bedtime routine** – not necessarily an easy task for parents as this can be a hectic time of the day with meals to prepare and older children needing attention. A warm bath, a final drink and a bedtime story (non-exciting) are ideal. This to be followed by a calm but firm tucking down and saying 'Good night'. Requests for 'a drink', 'to come downstairs' need to be firmly resisted. Once given in to, the pattern can be hard to break. This can be especially difficult following an illness where the child has obvious reasons for being unable to sleep. Any illness, of course, will need specific and appropriate treatment.

Night-time waking can be due to any number of causes, and efforts will need to be made to sort out the individual reasons for the waking. Perhaps the child is disturbed by a specific noise at some time of the night? Or perhaps the lack of general household noise during the evening is a factor? It is surprising how comforting sounds of activity in other parts of the house can be when dropping off to sleep. A **night-light**, or landing or hall light left on, can reassure a child who wakes for some reason during the night. Again, any possible illness will need to be found and treated.

Nightmares need reassurance that the unpleasant experience was only a dream and not a reality. A cuddle and the continuing **presence of an adult** until the child sleeps again is all that is needed. Recurrent nightmares should alert parents to the fact that there is some factor in the child's daily life that is causing concern. Maybe some activity or recurring events at nursery or school needs explanation or alteration. Every individual child will react in a different way to the day-to-day events of everyday life.

Night terrors can be more difficult to handle. Again, identifying **potential stressful activities** during the day can help. Parents also find it reassuring to know that the child has no recollection of the night-time fears. Children with night terrors will eventually grow out of these experiences.

Sleep-walkers need to be **protected from injuring themselves** during their perambulations – for example, gently guiding them away from stairs or pieces of heavy furniture that could cause injury. They should be led back to bed without any attempt being made to wake them. Sleep walking occurs during the phase of deepest sleep and waking in a strange, unexpected place can be frightening. Any anxieties during the day need to be unearthed and discussed with the child.

THE FUTURE

Sleep problems by no means affect all children. Those that do, however, give parents cause for much concern – and weariness! It is reassuring to be told that most sleep difficulties will be overcome by late childhood. There is no evidence to show that children with sleep problems have similar difficulties in later life.

SQUINT

ALTERNATIVE NAME

Strabismus. While squints in children are not a disease entity like, for example, an infectious condition or a congenital problem, early treatment is vital if full vision is to be preserved.

INCIDENCE

The exact incidence of squints in children is not documented. But it is thought that around 50% of children who do have a squint have someone else in the family who has the same condition. The squint itself is not directly inherited, but the factors that are associated with the production of the squint can be passed on from generation to generation. In view of this, it is important that the brothers and sisters of a child with a squint should also be examined for this condition.

It is especially important to diagnose those children in whom the squint is not immediately obvious. Small or latent squints can have as great a deleterious effect on good binocular vision as can a more obvious squint.

Squints can occur in any axis of the eye. But by far the commonest types of squint are the **convergent** type (in which one eye is seen to turn inwards) and the **divergent** type (in which one eye is seen to turn outwards).

All babies squint at times for the first few weeks after birth before muscle co-ordination is fully developed. But any squint in a baby over the age of 4 months should be investigated.

CAUSATION

There are a number of conditions which can be factors in the aetiology of a squint.

- A **refractive error in one eye** is by far the commonest cause of a squint. Under these circumstances, one eye focuses clearly on an object at a different distance from the other eye. For example, a convergent squint can occur when one eye focuses clearly on an object at a greater distance away than does the other eye. (This is known as hypermetropia.) To pull these two perceived objects into one image, the 'long distance' seeing eye will need to accommodate (be pulled by the eye muscles into the right position) to a greater extent than the other eye. Conversely, a short-sighted (myopic) eye – focusing clearly on nearer objects – will need less accommodation, and so a divergent squint will be the result.

- **Injuries to the cornea**, resulting in scarring of this external sensitive part of the eye, can also give rise to a squint. This has a similar effect to that produced by a short-sighted eye, in as much as vision in the damaged eye is reduced.
- The onset of a squint in a previously non-squinting child can also be the first clue to **diseases of the retina or optic nerve**, such as, for example, a retinoblastoma.
- **Occlusion of one eye** by a pad or bandage, following some injury to an eye or the face, can cause a squint to develop in a surprisingly short time. The covered eye will become non-seeing, or 'amblyopic', through disuse. Treatment to reverse this process must be undertaken with a degree of urgency to prevent permanent loss of vision in this eye.

While a simple refractive error is the commonest cause of a squint, the other possible factors must always be borne in mind.

CHARACTERISTICS

Squints, as mentioned previously, come in a variety of guises – convergent or divergent and also, to a much lesser extent, in the vertical axis. Children with squints in the vertical axis will often tilt their heads to compensate for the squint – a useful clue that a squint may be present, although not immediately obvious.

As well as these differences in direction, squints can be alternating in character, i.e. one eye being fixed on an object at one time, only to be quickly followed by the other eye being fixed on the object instead. In this condition, true binocular vision (in which the two eyes fix and focus on one object to produce one image) is never achieved.

Squints can cause two images to be seen, although there is only one object (double vision). This is obviously not a situation that can continue! So the part of the brain concerned with vision will suppress one of these images – from a squinting eye, for example. As a knock-on result of this the eye will eventually lose all ability to see. This condition is known as **amblyopia**. It is to prevent this loss of vision in one eye that early intervention in squints is vital, as without treatment the lack of vision can become permanent.

Squints can be very obvious, even to the casual observer, or can be so small as to be virtually undetectable without special tests. It is important that observations by parents on their child's possible squint should not be dismissed but investigated fully.

A 'pseudo-squint' is often seen in children who have especially marked folds of skin (epicanthic folds) over the near side of their eyes. These skin folds can give the appearance of a squint by obscuring more of the white of the eye on the inner side. Specific tests (see below) will differentiate this effect from a true squint. This condition is more commonly noticed in younger children before the development of definite strong facial features.

Similar effects can also occur in children who have a broad bridge to their nose, or who have an asymmetrical face for some reason. Again, special tests will differentiate this.

A **latent squint** can become obvious when a child is ill with some intercurrent infection. Muscle control at this time is imperfect and a squint can be clearly seen. On recovery the squint will disappear, but if this is noticed it is as well to check with an orthoptist that there is no squint.

Squints are not caused by anxiety, fear or infectious disease, as some 'old wives' tales' would have us believe.

INVESTIGATIONS

- **Tests for refractive errors.** These will include tests for short-sight, long-sight and astigmatism, with special reference to differences in the two eyes. (An astigmatism occurs when the lens of the eye is less than perfectly shaped, so that distorted images bounce off this ill-shaped refractive surface.)
- **Examination of light reflexes.** Shining a light, from a pencil torch for example, into the child's eye will show whether or not the reflection from the light occurs in the same position in each eye. If, for example, the light is reflected to the right of the pupil in one eye and over the pupil in the other, some degree of squint is present.
- **The 'cover test'.** This test involves covering one of the child's eyes with a hand, or card, while the child is focusing on a distant object. On removal of the cover, the covered eye will be seen to move if a squint is present. If there is no squint, neither eye will move on taking away the covering hand or card. This test should be repeated two or three times in quick succession.
- **Orthoptic tests**, with special equipment, to measure the angle of the squint can be carried out once the presence of a definite squint has been established.
- **Full examination by an ophthalmologist**, with the eyes fully dilated, is necessary when causes other than simple refractive errors are suspected. This is vital to exclude serious eye disease.

MANAGEMENT

- **Correction of any refractive error** is the first essential. This involves routine tests, appropriate to the age of the child, for long- or short-sight as well as for an astigmatism. Spectacles are then pre-scribed to correct these errors. In many cases this will result in an im-provement of the squint. It will be necessary to constantly review the strength of the visual correction. With growth, the refractive errors in a long-sighted child can improve so much that the spectacles can be discarded at a later date.
- **Occlusion of the good eye** for 1 or 2 weeks at a time may be necessary to obtain good vision in the squinting eye. This is often necessary if a degree of amblyopia has developed in the squinting eye.

- **Orthoptic exercises** are also valuable in producing good binocular vision.
- If the above treatments are not adequate, **surgery** can be necessary to correct the squint. This is carried out under a general anaesthetic. The muscles moving the eyes are then lengthened, shortened or repositioned according to the type and degree of the squint.
- Occasionally, instillation of **eye-drops** that cause accommodation of the squinting eye to decrease have been used with success in small angle squints.
- Other, more recent and experimental, treatments have been used to induce a temporary, partial **paralysis** of the eye-muscles. This allows time for binocular vision to become established.

THE FUTURE

Amblyopia can occur if a squint remains undiagnosed and untreated for some time. Amblyopia becomes of great importance to the person if, at a late date, vision is lost in the normally seeing eye. Full vision can never be fully restored to an amblyopic eye.

SELF-HELP GROUPS

Royal National Institute for the Blind (RNIB)
224 Great Portland Street
London, W1N 6AA
Tel. 0171 388 1266.

The Partially Sighted Society
62 Salusbury Road
London, NW6 6NS
Tel. 0171 372 1551.

It is to be hoped that no child with a simple squint will ever need to be in contact with either of the above societies. Only if the squint is an early manifestation of some other ocular disease should severe visual handicap be a problem.

STERNOMASTOID TUMOUR

ALTERNATIVE NAMES

Torticollis; wry neck. (These names are not true alternatives, as there are a number of other causes of torticollis. For example, a development abnormality in one of the vertebrae in the neck or a severe lymph node infection will give rise to a similar picture. Both these alternative names are, however, frequently applied to the condition.)

INCIDENCE

The incidence of this relatively mild condition has not been reported, but clinically it seems to appear with a fair degree of regularity in surgeries and clinics. It is more common in babies who have had a breech birth. Boys and girls are equally affected.

CAUSATION

Again, this is unknown, but the relationship between a breech birth and a sternomastoid tumour is well documented. Originally it was thought to be due to the trauma of a breech delivery. More recently, however, it seems likely that the abnormality exists prenatally and is possibly the cause – and not the outcome – of breech birth.

CHARACTERISTICS

The basic abnormality is in one of the sternomastoid muscles in the neck. These muscles link the bony mastoid process behind the ear to the top of the sternum. Their important function is the turning of the head. With a sternomastoid tumour, part of the muscular tissue of this structure has been replaced by fibrous tissue, which effectively reduces the turn of the head. In no way is this abnormality dangerous to health or likely to spread to any other part of the body. Usually it is around 2–3 weeks of age that the condition is noticed by the parents. Their baby is seen to be **continually looking upwards** and with the **head tilted** to one side. On examining the neck, a **hard swelling** is found in one of the sternomastoid muscles.

MANAGEMENT

Physiotherapy needs to be started as soon as possible after diagnosis. Exercises consist of gently rotating the baby's head to stretch the affected muscle.

Surgery may be required if the condition is missed in early life or if treatment fails to achieve a satisfactory result. Without adequate treatment the child's face and neck will develop asymmetrically as well as causing possible involvement of the underlying structures in the neck.

The future

With adequate and successful treatment there are no deleterious after-effects from a sternomastoid tumour.

Sudden infant death syndrome (SIDS)

Alternative name

Cot death.

Incidence

The incidence of this tragic event varies widely between countries and over time. In the UK during the 1980s the incidence was between 1.6 and 2.2 for every 1000 babies born. This meant that approximately 1500 babies died every year from this cause. In Hong Kong the incidence was much lower – 0.2 for every 1000 live births, while in New Zealand the incidence was higher – 3–4 babies for every 1000 born. No satisfactory explanation of these differences has been given.

Since the late 1980s much attention and research has been directed towards possible causes and ways of prevention of SIDS. This has resulted in a dramatic decrease in the number of babies found unexpectedly dead in their cots. In the UK the incidence has dropped to 0.7 for every 1000 live births – a fall to approximately 450 deaths every year. A similar drop in incidence has also occurred in New Zealand.

A number of other features are of importance when looking at the incidence of cot death. The commonest age for this tragedy to occur is between 2 and 3 months of age. Very few deaths due to this cause occur in the first 2 weeks of life and after 7 months of age the danger is lessened, only around 10% of deaths occurring after this age.

Boys are more likely than girls to die in this way.

There is also a seasonal incidence, with more deaths happening in the winter months. (Possibly this has something to do with the higher incidence of upper respiratory tract infections at this time of the year? A small proportion of babies were found to have had symptoms of a mild viral infection in the days immediately before death.)

SIDS occurs in all socioeconomic groups, but there appears to be an increased risk with deprivation – and also with women who have borne many children, young mothers and low-birthweight babies.

From all these facts it is likely that there are a number of causative factors involved in the unexpected death of a young baby.

History

The sudden unexpected death syndrome has been described from time immemorial. It was usual in those far-off days to put this down to 'over-laying' or a deliberate act on the part of one or other parent.

('Over-laying' was the term applied to the supposed suffocation of the baby by parents – often thought to be drunk – rolling over on to the baby sleeping in the same bed.) It was only during the latter half of the 20th century, when more babies slept by themselves in cots, that it became clear that sudden unexpected death did occur for reasons other than over-laying. But these reasons were unknown in spite of detailed post-mortem examination.

CAUSATION

As mentioned previously, there is no one known factor that can be definitely associated with a cot death. There are, however, a number of practices in the care of young babies which have resulted in the fall of the incidence of this devastating condition.

- **Sleeping position of the baby.** It is advised that babies are laid to sleep on their backs or on their sides and not face downwards – the supine (or face upwards) position being preferable to the side position. This simple practice appears to be the most important action in reducing the number of babies suffering a cot death.
- **Tobacco smoke.** Parents – and visitors – are advised not to smoke anywhere where there is a young baby. Also, mothers are advised not to smoke at all during pregnancy. Exposure to tobacco smoke is considered to be the single largest potentially avoidable factor in SIDS. (As well as having a bearing on the incidence of cot death, children raised in non-smoking households have fewer upper respiratory tract infections that those children whose parents smoke.)
- **Overheating** has been suggested as a possible cause for cot death. With today's centrally heated homes, babies do not need warm night clothes and multiple bed coverings at night. A nursery thermometer is a good guide to the temperature of the room where the baby sleeps, so that bedclothes can adjusted accordingly. Duvets and baby nests especially can create an extremely warm environment, and it must be remembered that babies cannot move and throw off excess coverings if they feel too hot.
- **Breast-fed babies** appear to be less at risk of cot death than babies fed on formula milk. It is possible that some form of allergy may be a factor here.
- **Mild infection** is thought also to be a possible factor, although many babies with infections survive these with no problems. Parents, however, are advised to contact their doctor if they are at all worried about their young baby's health – particularly under the age of 7 months.
- Regrettably, **non-accidental injury** must always be remembered as a cause of cot death.

Careful and sensitive handling at this traumatic time is vital.

Management

In this context, 'management' refers to the sequence of actions needing to be taken after the discovery of the unexpected death of a baby. The parents' first contact will be either their own general practitioner or the accident and emergency department of the local hospital after their devastating finding. The baby will be examined and parents asked to remember, if possible, the sequence of events that led up to the time when they found their baby dead. This should include any worries they may have had regarding the baby's health the day or two before.

It is important that parents are given the chance to hold their dead baby, as this does much to aid the normal grieving process. It is necessary in all instances of cot death that the coroner (or in Scotland the Procurator Fiscal) is informed and a **post-mortem examination** carried out. This can seem unnecessary – and upsetting – for parents, but it is important that any known cause of death is identified. Relatives and/or **friends should be contacted** before the parents return home, and a **medical social worker** can be of comfort and support at this time.

An information leaflet from the Foundation for the Study of Infant Deaths will give sympathetic and accurate information to parents who always wish to know exactly what has happened to their baby. Later contact can be arranged, if the parents wish, with local **cot death parental support**.

It is also important that parents are given a chance to **discuss events** 2–3 weeks later with the paediatrician involved at the time of their baby's death. Many anxieties and queries will have arisen over this time that need discussion and clarification.

At a later date, if a **further pregnancy** is considered, parents will need much support. Fears of a recurrence are always uppermost when caring for a young baby again. An organization – under the banner of the Foundation for the Study of Infant Deaths – called CONI (Care of the Next Infant) gives advice and support at this time.

Prevention

At present, factors that have reduced the incidence of SIDS are:

- babies put to sleep **face upwards**;
- **avoidance of tobacco smoke** – both before and after birth;
- **avoidance of overheating**;
- **breast-feed** if possible;
- check carefully on minor episodes of **illness** at the critical ages.

The future

Research is continuing in many parts of the world on all aspects of the sudden infant death syndrome.

SELF-HELP GROUP

Foundation for the Study of Infant Deaths (FSID)
14 Halkin Street
London, SW1X 7DP
Tel. 0171 235 0965
Cot death helpline (24-hour) 0171 235 1721.

TEMPER TANTRUMS

INCIDENCE

Probably every child has had at least one temper tantrum in the early years of life – perhaps mild only, but nevertheless a temper tantrum! These can be isolated incidents or can occur more frequently as part of wider behaviour problems.

Both sexes seem to be equally affected, and the usual age group affected is between 18 months and 3–4 years.

CAUSATION

Between the ages of 18 months and 3 years children's verbal and physical skills are developing fast. So also are their desires to handle objects, behave in a more 'grown-up' way and attempt tasks beyond their physical competence. It is when these two facets of development do not agree that a temper tantrum can result. **Frustration**, or just plain **hurting themselves** when attempting a too difficult task, can be precipitating factors.

From a wider viewpoint, outside factors can be involved in the frequency and severity of a temper tantrum. **Physical disability** or **chronic illness** can give rise to greater degrees of frustration. The child sees peers behaving in a way that highlights his/her disability – a potent reason for venting anger.

Parental difficulties, such as marital disharmony or parental illness for example, can all have profound effects on a child's perceptions and reactions. In an attempt to gain security, a temper tantrum may be the only way possible for a child to express feelings. Poverty or other forms of **social deprivation**, including poor parenting skills, can have a similar effect.

A child's specific **temperament** will also have a bearing on the range of the temper tantrums. The quiet, easy-going child will feel no need to express him/herself in this way. Other children with more outgoing, and perhaps more aggressive, personalities will be more prone to these outbursts.

CHARACTERISTICS

These can vary widely, but everyone has seen, and felt sympathy for, the young mother struggling with a load of shopping and a toddler lying on the floor of the supermarket screaming and kicking. The more aggressive-natured children will fly at siblings or parents and attack them physically – but only very rarely hurting themselves in the process!

Breath-holding attacks are a specific – and frightening – form of temper tantrum. Again, they are usually precipitated by anger, frustration or an emotional upset. The child cries for a few minutes and then holds the breath and stops breathing. The face will turn blue and, on occasions, consciousness will be lost and the child falls to the ground. Jerking movements of the limbs can follow and it is a difficult decision to decide whether or not this is an epileptic fit or a simple breath-holding attack. With a breath-holding attack, however, recovery is quick and complete, whereas the child who has had a fit will be drowsy and confused for a time.

Somewhat similar, but even more alarming, are **reflex anoxic seizures**. Here the child becomes suddenly extremely pale and limp, and consciousness is lost. Recovery is rapid – within 1 minute – and complete. Again, this event can follow on from some minor injury such as a bumped head or a scratched knee. These attacks are due to the overactivity of a specific nerve in control of the pulse. There is often a familial tendency to these worrying attacks.

MANAGEMENT

Most temper tantrums are self limiting, the child ceasing the antisocial activity and starting to sob or cry quietly. It is important that parents should recognize their child's need for reassurance and affection at this time. (This can be a difficult task considering the difficulties in which the child has put parents just a few minutes earlier!) But it must be remembered that the child, too, is overwhelmed by previous feelings of anger or frustration and can feel very frightened at the strength of the emotions experienced.

It can be necessary to **restrain a child** in the throes of a temper tantrum, because of the possible physical danger to themselves or other people. The best way to do this is to fold arms around the child's body from behind and so stop flailing arms and legs from creating mayhem. A further difficult task is to avoid excess attention to the child in a tantrum! – rather must praise be given when behaviour is good.

Breath-holding attacks and **reflex anoxic seizures** need to be **discussed with a doctor**, particularly if twitching of the limbs has occurred during these attacks. It is important to distinguish between these attacks and an epileptic seizure. A good description of the events before the attack can be helpful in clarifying the diagnosis.

Reflex anoxic seizures may continue throughout early childhood and can be frequent. Treatment with **atropine** has been found to be effective if these occurrences are too frequent, but this must be prescribed by the child's doctor.

THE FUTURE

Temper tantrums are usually grown out of by the time school days start, coinciding with children's increased ability to express themselves and their feelings.

Reflex Anoxic Seizure Group (RAS)
PO Box 175
Stratford-on-Avon, CV37 8YD
Tel. 01789 450564.

THREADWORM

ALTERNATIVE NAMES

Pin worm; seat worm.

INCIDENCE

Threadworms are common throughout the world and are – surprisingly – especially common in countries with a colder climate. The age group most often affected are boys and girls between the ages of 5 and 9 years – the primary school years. (Research in the late 1980s suggests that there is a further peak in incidence between the ages of 30 and 49 years. Possibly this is because this is the age group who most frequently live with children in the 5–9-year age group and so are infected along with their children?)

Infestation occurs more commonly in urban areas. It is thought that up to 50% of London children are infested with threadworms at any one time.

CAUSATION

Infestation with threadworms is passed on from child to child by hand contact, or contact with soiled underclothes or bedlinen. The tiny eggs of the threadworm are laid, in many thousands, around the child's anus during sleep. These eggs can then be transferred on fingers, following scratching, to the mouth. The eggs than hatch on the way through the intestine. The adult worms then mate and the female again lays further thousands of eggs and the cycle is repeated.

Spread is by the minute eggs being passed on to others from the dust in the bedlinen or by contact with soiled bed- or underclothes. The eggs can survive in dust, at room temperature, for up to 2 or 3 weeks.

Domestic animals, of any kind, play no part in the dissemination of threadworms. This differs from the mode of spread of other worms.

CHARACTERISTICS

Over the years, threadworms have been thought of as causing many symptoms in children – nail-biting, convulsions and hyperactivity, to mention just a few. None of these conditions are due to threadworms.

Irritation around the anus can be due to the presence of the worm. It is also possible that **sleep can be disturbed** by the presence of the egg-laying worm. Some authorities also consider that **bed-wetting** can be due to this cause. In girls, **irritation around the vulval area** can result from infestation with threadworms.

Parents can also, at times, be alarmed to see worms in their child's stools. This does not occur, however, as frequently as would be expected because of the smallness of the worm – only around 10 mm long.

INVESTIGATIONS

The best method to determine whether or not a child is infested with threadworms is to wrap a piece of Sellotape (sticky side out) around a test-tube or spatula and apply this to the child's anus. The tape is then transferred to a microscope slide. The eggs, if present, can readily be seen when the slide is visualized under the microscope. (The child should not have bathed or had bowels open before this test is performed.) It may be necessary to repeat this investigation for three consecutive days as the worms do not necessarily pass through the intestine in a regular manner.

MANAGEMENT

There are a number of **drugs** that will effectively eliminate threadworms. Usually only one dose is needed. It is advisable that all members of the family should be treated, because of the many thousands of eggs that can be present in the bedlinen and the general household dust.

Hygiene, especially in personal cleanliness, is vital in controlling infestations with threadworms. Children should be taught the importance of **hand-washing** before meals and after visiting the toilet. **Fingernails** should be cut short to reduce the possibility of the eggs remaining in this situation. Frequent changes of underwear and bedlinen are also of importance in the control of infestation with threadworms.

Parents will also need **reassurance** that they are not alone in having threadworms as visitors to their family, and, secondly, that their child will not suffer permanent harm.

COMPLICATIONS

Very occasionally there may be such a heavy infestation of threadworms in the bowel that the child may complain of **abdominal pain**. This will be cured by the appropriate treatment to eliminate the worms. (Threadworms have been found in the lumen of the appendix following removal of this organ, but it is not thought that this has any bearing on the onset of the appendicitis.)

PREVENTION

This is limited to good personal hygiene and prompt and adequate treatment of the whole family if an infestation is found to be present.

Tics

Alternative names

Habit disorder; habit spasm.

Incidence

It is thought that the rapid, repetitive, involuntary muscular movements known as habit spasms affect as many as 10% of the childhood population at any one time. Children between the ages of 7 and 12 years are most commonly affected. Boys outnumber girls three to one in these habits. There is frequently a family history of habit spasms. A proportion of habit spasms do persist into adult life.

History

A variety of bizarre tics have been described in literature – Dickens being the master of this.

Causation

Frequently, a **stressful home or school situation** can be found in a child who has a tic. It would seem that the tic has been developed almost as a superstitious ritual against the stress in these circumstances. **Imitation** is also a powerful stimulus to the development of a tic. A schoolfellow with twitchy eyes, or a grandfather with a limp, can often be found in the child's immediate environment.

Differentiation of simple tics from chorea and the Gilles de la Tourette syndrome must be made. In **chorea** (a symptom seen in a number of illnesses, including a type of cerebral palsy, or following encephalitis, for example) the movements are not so stereotyped and predictable as with habit spasms. **Gilles de la Tourette syndrome** is a particularly distressing ailment where there are many violent, complex muscular tics associated frequently with the repetition of obscene words and an odd form of barking cough. This syndrome is extremely difficult to treat and can continue into adult life in around 50% of cases – a differential point with common tics.

Characteristics

Tics can affect any part of the body, but are most usually seen to involve the head and neck areas. **Blinking** of the eyes, **twisting of the mouth** and/or **shrugging of the shoulders** are among the commonest tics noted.

It is always the **same group of muscles** that are involved in each series of movements, so that one is aware in advance of exactly what will be happening next. (This is in direct contradistinction to involuntary movements due to other physical causes.)

Repetitive coughing, swallowing or sneezing are other – irritating! – forms of tic found in children. These tics often begin under circumstances of acute embarrassment for the child, and continue when the particular stress is removed.

MANAGEMENT

Most cases of habit spasm resolve spontaneously given time. But it is thought that about 6% of children with tics will still have their specific habit spasm as adults.

Parents should be advised **not to grumble at or ridicule** their child with a tic. This is counterproductive and only draws attention to the problem.

Family therapy can help where there are family tensions and anxieties. General practitioners will be able to give advice on where and how to contact skilled people to undertake this therapy. **Behaviour therapy** is also helpful. Therapists can help parents on techniques to distract the child's attention when the tic is manifest.

Tranquillizers are a last resort to be tried, particularly if the child is overactive in addition to having a tic. These drugs must be carefully controlled, however, and never continued for any length of time.

THE FUTURE

The majority of simple tics resolve themselves by the time the teenage years are reached. A few adults will still have their tics throughout their lives, and these will become part of their individual personalities.

Tics caused by chorea or the Gilles de la Tourette syndrome have a less successful outcome and need specialized treatment.

There is a specific self-help group for parents of children with the Gilles de la Tourette syndrome:

SELF-HELP GROUP

Tourette Syndrome (UK) Association
Valley Mead
27 Monkton Street
Ryde
Isle of Wight, PO33 2BY
Tel. 01983 568866.

Tonsillitis

Incidence

As tonsillitis is not a notifiable condition, there are no figures available as to this unpleasant infection of the throat so common in children. But all doctor's surgeries – especially during the winter months – will see several children every week with tonsillitis. Preschool and early school-age children usually suffer from three or four upper respiratory infections during the course of any one year. While all these infections are by no means tonsillitis, a significant number of these infections will involve these pads of lymphatic tissue – the 'watch-dogs' of the throat. (Anatomically the pharynx, housing the tonsils at either side, is closely allied to the middle ear. Infection frequently occurs in both these parts of the body simultaneously – but for descriptive purposes it is best that they are discussed separately.)

Boys and girls are affected equally, and tonsillitis is seen in all races.

Causation

The tonsils are two masses of lymphoid tissue situated at the back of the throat, and in children they are relatively large up to the age of 8 years – even when clear of infection. They fulfil the function of dealing with bacteria and viruses before these invaders have the chance to proceed to the lower respiratory tract – the lungs and associated structures. As the tonsils perform their work dealing with infection, they become red and swollen. During this process, pain is felt and there is also a generalized constitutional upset.

Tonsillitis can be caused by either bacteria or viruses. It is impossible to determine which infecting organism is causing the symptoms without laboratory confirmation from a swab of the child's throat.

Characteristics

Fever is one of the first and most common signs of tonsillitis. In young children in particular this can be high, and can give rise to a febrile convulsion. (These are convulsions caused by the reaction of the immature brain to a high body temperature. They rarely occur after the age of 5 years.)

A **sore throat** is more often complained of by older children than those in the under-5 bracket. These latter children frequently complain of a '**tummy-ache**' rather than a sore throat. In both age-groups there will a **reluctance to eat**.

On looking down the throat of the sufferer, the cause of the problem will become obvious. The tonsils are **red and swollen**. In really severe infections, the two tonsils are seen to almost meet in the mid-line of the throat – causing no surprise that the child is refusing food!

Swollen glands in the neck are also a frequent feature of tonsillitis. These cervical glands drain infection from the back of the throat, and in so doing become enlarged and tender. A **blocked, stuffy nose** can also accompany an infection in the tonsils. This is due to associated infection in the adenoids – masses of lymphoid tissue situated at the back of the nose. These tissues also become swollen and inflamed by the infective process.

The child with tonsillitis will feel generally **unwell** and miserable.

INVESTIGATIONS

Tonsillitis is diagnosed by the clinical signs and symptoms. Theoretically, a throat swab sent to the laboratory will determine the causative infective organism. In practice this is rarely done, as treatment needs to be started before the laboratory results become available.

MANAGEMENT

The acute attack

Penicillin is the antibiotic of first choice for an attack of tonsillitis, and will relieve unpleasant symptoms within 24–48 hours. It is important, however, that the full course that has been prescribed should be taken, in order to fully eradicate the invading organism. **Paracetamol** (in doses and strengths appropriate to the age of the child) should be given – at 4-hourly intervals, if necessary initially – to relieve sore throat and headache. This drug will also help to lower the temperature.

Fluids only for the first 24–48 hours of the infection will be all that the young sufferer will be willing to take. It is vital that sufficient fluid is given at this time. Children can quickly become dehydrated as a result of the high fever so frequently seen during an acute attack of tonsillitis.

Bed-rest is not essential, unless the child feels more comfortable tucked up in bed. Quiet play in a warm room with the chance to lie down on occasions is usually a favoured option for a young child with an acute attack of tonsillitis.

Tonsillectomy

This operation has had its fashionable periods, tonsils being very readily removed for slight reasons in bygone days. Today's criteria for this operation are more rigid. Most ear, nose and throat surgeons would only consider removing a child's tonsils if:

- the child has suffered from more than three attacks of confirmed tonsillitis in 1 year over a 2-year period; and/or
- the tonsils are so large as to meet in the mid-line even when an acute infection is not present. This state of affairs can be dangerous to normal breathing, especially during sleep.

Tonsillectomy is performed by an ear, nose and throat surgeon under a general anaesthetic. At this time the surgeon will also consider whether or not removal of the adenoids is necessary. A stay of one or two nights in hospital is the general rule. Children recover very quickly from the removal of their tonsils – far more rapidly than do adults undergoing this procedure. Cool fluids and a soft, easy-to-swallow diet for a day or two is all that is needed by way of postoperative care. For school-age children, a couple of weeks off school is advisable to ensure that further throat infections are not contracted too soon after the operation.

THE FUTURE

If a child's tonsils have been chronically infected for a number of years, with frequent attacks of acute infection, s/he will be seen to benefit enormously from tonsillectomy. Appetite, energy and general well-being will all improve and growth will often show a spurt. On the down side, however, the mere fact of having had a tonsillectomy does not mean that sore throats are a thing of the past! Throat infections can – and do – still occur. But these are less frequent and recovery is quicker in the child whose tonsils had been a source of chronic infection.

Toxocara

Incidence

The incidence of infections with toxocara – a type of roundworm – is not precisely known. Infections with this parasite may be more than is recognized – the child's immunity being built up before the condition is diagnosed.

Causation

The *Toxocara canis* worm is a normal inhabitant of the intestine of the young dog and the fox. These animals gain natural immunity to the parasite by around 6 months of age, and the adult worms are then expelled from their bodies at this time – so no ill effects are seen in older dogs, although the worms may still exist in an encapsulated form. But during pregnancy, bitches lose this immunity. Reinfection, or reactivation of the dormant larvae occurs, thereby affecting the unborn puppies. So, at birth, these puppies are infected with the toxocara worm.

Children acquire the infection by swallowing the minute eggs of toxocara – either directly from the tongues of the puppies when they are licked, or from crawling around on carpets, lawns and other areas where eggs may be deposited. As would be expected, younger children – during the crawling years especially – are the most frequently affected age group. At this age, too, exploration of everyday objects is largely done by taking them to the mouth. When inside the child's body the larvae (arising from the ingested eggs) are unable to mature in the child's intestine – where, in the dog and fox, they normally find their home. So they wander aimlessly around the child's body, setting up areas of inflammation in a variety of sites – liver, kidneys, lungs, muscles, brain and eyes can all be possibly affected. (This wandering is known by the splendidly descriptive name of 'visceral larvae migrans'.) It is also thought that the type of toxocara affecting cats – *Toxocara catis* – causes similar symptoms.

Characteristics

Signs and symptoms of infection with toxocara can be very diverse. The diagnosis of infection with toxocara may never be made as the child has such a possible wide variety of non-specific symptoms and may recover spontaneously. However, certain clues can help.

- The age of the child affected is usually between 1 and 7 years – the early years of crawling and putting many different objects into the mouth. At this age, also, hygiene is rudimentary!

- There is frequently the arrival in the home of a new puppy prior to the onset of symptoms.

Signs and symptoms of infection can include:

- **failure to thrive adequately**, i.e. poor weight gain and lack of general growth;
- a liking of eating all kinds of strange substances (earth, coal); this is known as **pica**;
- a **low-grade fever**;
- a **cough**, with episodes of wheezing;
- **anaemia**;
- **convulsions**;
- **blurring of vision** with possible subsequent loss of vision due to involvement of the retina.

The blurring is caused by inflammation of this vital part of the eye, and the possible subsequent loss of vision is caused by the detachment of the retina. Children with these ocular manifestations tend to be in the older age group – between 7 and 9 years.

Not all these symptoms, of course, occur in any one infected child. The symptoms will depend on which organ, or system of the body, is involved in the infection.

Untreated, the infection runs a slow, benign course with the child's natural defence mechanisms eventually overcoming the infection. Usually within 18 months, full health is restored.

INVESTIGATIONS

Blood tests will show if any anaemia is present, and can also be used for serological testing to determine if antibodies against toxocara are present. (It is interesting to note that up to 7% of adults show positive results to this latter test. This implies that they have been infected, at some time or other in their earlier life, by toxocara. No very obvious symptoms may have occurred – that can be remembered – but they have successfully overcome the infection.)

MANAGEMENT

Often the diagnosis of toxocara is uncertain for some time, and the child's very general and non-specific symptoms are treated empirically. For example, antibiotics are given for the cough and iron medication for the anaemia. These medicines will result in improvement in the child's general health, as there can be added infection in the respiratory tract and an iron deficient anaemia as a result of a poor appetite.

Once investigations have proved that infection with toxocara is present, there are several specific drugs that can be used with success, although treatment may take several weeks. Steroids can also be used to advantage to reduce the inflammation at various sites in the body.

COMPLICATIONS

The most serious complication is the loss of vision that can result from the migrating larvae in the eye. Again, there are specific drugs available, which are valuable in treating this condition and can help to preserve vision.

PREVENTION

Infection of children with toxocara has evoked much 'anti-dog' publicity over recent years. But two points must be remembered.

- Infections of all kinds abound in our immediate environs and toxocara is just one of them. With care and good hygiene this infection can be contained as readily – and more so – as many others.
- Pets of all kinds are valuable to both children and elderly people. Children learn care as they attend to their pets needs as well as learning facts about the animal creation. Lonely and upset children – of which there are regretfully many in our stressful society today – can gain much comfort from a pet.

A few sensible precautions will, however, need to be taken to ensure that the risk of Toxocara infection of young children is reduced to a minimum.

- Dogs should be wormed regularly with the appropriate medication – available from chemists or vets.
- Children should be taught not to allow dogs to lick their faces, and to wash their hands thoroughly after fondling their pets, and certainly always before eating.
- Dog owners should control their dogs at all times, and should not allow them to foul public walk-ways or open spaces.
- Communities should ensure that it is not possible for dogs to foul playing fields, sand-pits or other places where children are encouraged to play.

If these precautions are adhered to, toxocara infections could be eliminated without the need to destroy or ban all dogs as pets.

The following group gives information on ways of preventing Toxocara infection.

SELF-HELP GROUP

Community Hygiene Concern
32 Crane Avenue
Isleworth
Middlesex, TW7 7JL
Tel. 0181 341 7167.

TUBERCULOSIS

INCIDENCE

In developed countries of the world, tuberculosis (TB) has reduced rapidly in incidence over the past half century or so. In 1947, 2000 children died from tuberculosis in England and Wales. Forty years later, in the years between 1985 and 1987, just three children died from the disease. A dramatic reduction indeed. This fall is due to better living conditions and less overcrowding as well as better treatment of known cases of tuberculosis. 'Contact tracing', and subsequent treatment if necessary of people having lived or worked in close proximity to a sufferer, has also done much to reduce the incidence of tuberculosis. Nevertheless, this infectious disease remains an important problem in the UK, especially among immigrant peoples, particularly those from the Indian subcontinent. People living in unhygienic conditions are also at increased risk of contracting this disease.

Worldwide the picture is different. It is estimated that every year there are between 3 and 4 million infectious new cases of tuberculosis, with probably an equal number of people having smear-negative (or non-infectious) tuberculosis. The figure for children suffering from tuberculosis worldwide is around 1.25 million cases every year. Of these, 500 000 children will die from the disease.

(The difference between infectious and non-infectious cases of tuberculosis is important from the point of view of spread of the disease. Infectious cases are those people who cough up the infecting organism, which can thus be passed on to other people – children and adults. These people are known as 'smear-positive', as the offending bacteria can be isolated from their sputum. Non-infectious people can have the disease – in any number of systems of their bodies, including the lungs – but do not cough up the organism. They are therefore known as 'smear-negative', as their sputum does not contain the tuberculosis bacillus.

When infection with tuberculosis has occurred, the body becomes sensitive to the protein contained in the bacillus. This sensitivity shows itself in a positive skin reaction when a special preparation of the purified protein derivative (PPD) of the tuberculosis bacterium is injected into the superficial layers of the skin. This is the basis for the Mantoux, Heaf and Tine tests described below. Epidemiological data on the number of children showing a positive reaction in 1950 and in 1990 emphasizes further the decline in infection with tuberculosis. In 1950, almost 50% of the 14-year-old children tested were found to be positive – showing that they had met and overcome infection with tuberculosis bacteria. In 1990 less than 1% of children tested in a similar age group were found to be positive.)

CAUSATION

Tuberculosis is caused by a bacteria of the *Mycobacterium* genus, and was first described by Dr Robert Koch. As well as tuberculosis being passed on from other human beings, the infection can be transmitted in milk from infected cows. This mode of transmission never occurs in developed countries these days because all herds of dairy cows are tuberculin-tested to be sure that they are free from this disease.

CHARACTERISTICS

The initial infection with tuberculosis is in the lung. This **primary focus** can subsequently progress in two different ways.

On settling in the lungs, the bacteria will multiply here (usually in the upper part of one or other lung). The lymph nodes draining the affected part of the lung will also become involved in the infection. This group of involved tissues is then known as the **primary complex**. This infection can easily pass unnoticed, or occasionally the child will run a low-grade fever and be vaguely off-colour for a week or two. The body's natural defences are mobilized and seal off the infected area of lung. It is at this stage – which is reached within 4–6 weeks – that the skin tests for tuberculosis become positive. The lesion in the lung is usually too small to be visualized on X-ray, although the inflamed lymph nodes around the area can often be seen.

The primary infection that proceeds along these lines is not infectious to anyone else. Later in life this primary focus can become reactivated. The tuberculosis bacillus can remain dormant for many years. Symptoms can occur when the bacteria is released from its dormant position by a general lowering of the body's resistance for a variety of reasons – other illness or a general decline in health, for example.

The second type of progression occurs if the child is poorly nourished, ill with another intercurrent infection, taking immunosuppressant drugs for some other condition or merely in generally low health. Under these circumstances the initial infection with the tuberculosis bacteria can spread, through the blood, to a wide range of other tissues in the body, including further invasion of the lung.

In the lung, extensive destruction of lung tissue can result and the child will be seriously ill. There will be a **fever**, a **persistent cough** and **night sweats**. Fortunately this picture is rarely encountered in the UK today, but has always to be remembered in connection with this classic triad of symptoms.

The TB bacillus can invade the **meninges** (the delicate tissue covering the brain and spinal cord), giving rise to **tuberculous meningitis**. Symptoms of this will be the usual ones of meningitis due to any cause – headache, vomiting and fever. Lumbar puncture will obtain a sample of cerebrospinal fluid for laboratory analysis to determine the invading organism causing the symptoms.

Bone can also be affected by the spread of the bacteria. The spine is the most usual site affected, closely followed by knees and/or hips. The affected site will be painful, and X-ray changes will confirm the diagnosis.

Lymph-nodes, especially those in the neck, can also be the site to where the TB bacillus moves. Initially these infected glands will be enlarged but not tender as they are with a throat or ear infection. Later, if untreated, these swollen glands may break down and discharge. (Scars in this region of the neck are not infrequently seen in older people who have had to have these glands operated on.)

Other organs, e.g. **intestines, kidneys** and **larynx**, can be affected also, but these sites are rarely seen in children in western countries today.

All these latter aspects of spread from the primary focus are uncommon in developed countries of the world nowadays. But in other parts of the world, where poverty and disease are rife, these problems are not rare.

Investigations

X-ray of the chest, or other parts of the body where suspicious symptoms occur, will show in most cases the typical lesions of tuberculosis.

A **Heaf, Mantoux** or **Tine test** (described below) will also be positive if the infection is due to the tuberculosis bacterium. The extent of the reaction to these tests will point to the range of activity of the infection.

Management

The 'primary complex' is often not treated, as it frequently passes unnoticed. Even if the child is slightly feverish and off-colour for a short while, the true cause of the malaise is rarely discovered. Some authorities suggest that a known primary focus should be treated in order to prevent spread of the disease. (It must be emphasized that this primary focus is not infectious.)

Treatment for other forms of tuberculosis belong to a highly specialized area of medicine. There are a number of **drugs** available for use in tuberculosis infection today. (This is in direct contrast to bygone days when fresh air and good nutrition were the only available treatments.) These drugs will need to be continued for some length of time – up to 12–18 months in order to fully eradicate the disease. The child, of course, must be carefully monitored throughout this time, both for success of treatment and for possible adverse side-effects from the drugs used.

Attention to **living conditions** must also be of paramount importance in the successful management of tuberculosis. Adequate and appropriate **nutrition** of the sick child (and also probably the immediate family as well) can also need attention. Adequate **contact tracing** of other members of the family and other close social contacts must be carefully undertaken.

Schooling can be continued if the child feels well enough to cope with the demands of school. But arrangements for home tuition may well be necessary during the early stages of treatment, depending on the site and severity of the infection.

COMPLICATIONS

These have already been referred to in the generalized spread of tuberculosis.

PREVENTION

Prevention is by **immunization** with the Bacille Calmette–Guérin (BCG) vaccine. This was first produced by the Frenchmen Calmette and Guérin in 1921 – the vaccine being named after them. It was used in England to protect against the spread of tuberculosis from 1948 onwards.

In the UK, BCG immunization is recommended for four specific groups:

- newborn babies who live in households where there is a history of infection with the tuberculosis bacterium;
- babies born to immigrant families – people from the Indian subcontinent are particularly at risk, especially if return visits are made to India, where the infection is an ever-present problem;
- close contacts of people proved to be suffering from active tuberculosis;
- people whose work leads them into contact with possible sources of tuberculosis, such as health workers and students in teacher training colleges.

In addition to these groups, many authorities give BCG vaccine to all schoolchildren between the ages of 11 and 13 years. This procedure is regularly under review, as some authorities consider that good contact tracing, followed by either treatment or vaccination, is a preferable way of controlling the spread of infection.

Before the BCG vaccine is given a Heaf test is performed (the Mantoux test is similar but rarely used today – and the Tine test is used in younger children for its ease of use) 1 week to 10 days previously. This test involves introducing intradermally (usually by means of a special instrument with tiny prongs – the Heaf 'gun') a tiny amount of attenuated tuberculin. This test is done on the inside of the child's arm. The results are read a week later, and graded according to response from 0 to 4: 0 is equivalent to no response and 4 is equivalent to a reaction over 10 mm in diameter. Grade 2 readings and upwards imply that the child has met the tuberculosis bacillus and has developed immunity. Under these conditions the BCG vaccine will not need to be given. Children with grades 0 and 1 response will need immunization. As mentioned previously, the vast majority of children in the UK today show this latter reaction.

The BCG vaccination is given intradermally into the upper arm. This will result in a small spot within 2–4 weeks. Sometimes this can ulcerate and discharge, taking up to 3 months to finally heal. Contraindications to receiving the BCG vaccine are those children who have a malignancy or an immunological disease, or those children who are on steroids for some reason.

Tuberculosis is an infection against which vigilance must be maintained. In many parts of the world it is still a potent killer, and especially so of late in people with HIV infection. Rapid and adequate tracing of contacts of all cases of known tuberculosis is the first line of defence, with BCG vaccination a close second.

THE FUTURE

Old tuberculosis infection in the lung can be **reactivated** in later life if, for some reason, the body's defences are reduced. This could be a result of adverse physical surroundings, for example, or other illness or infection. It is vital that both the sufferers and their immediate contacts should receive quick and appropriate treatment.

Urinary tract infection

Incidence

Urinary tract infections are more common in childhood than used to be thought a few decades ago. Part of the reason for this is that the signs and symptoms are often so non-specific and intermittent that the problem is not diagnosed.

The prevalence is estimated to be between 1 and 2% in girls, but below 1% in boys. (In infancy this sex difference does not seem to apply – with as many boys being affected as girls.) It is thought that each general practice (of an average of around 10,000 people of all ages) will see at least two or three children every year with a new urinary tract infection. Perhaps this does not seem an enormous number, but for the individual child it is important that the diagnosis is made and the condition treated adequately to prevent further problems in later life.

Urinary tract infections can be the first clue given as to the presence of **abnormalities in the renal tract**. These abnormalities if undiscovered – and hence untreated – can again give rise to problems later in life.

Causation

Urinary tract infections are caused by bacteria. The type of bacteria involved are usually those found normally in the gastrointestinal tract where they do no harm. The *E. coli* bacteria is one of the most common types involved. Infection of the renal tract is usually prevented by the natural defence mechanisms of the body. For example, any bacteria gaining access to the bladder are regularly washed out by the flow of urine. Also, the child's natural immune defences preclude the infection gaining a hold in the renal tract. (Girls are more at risk from this method of infection than are boys due to the relative shortness of their urethra.) Breakdown of the natural defence mechanism can be caused by urine remaining in the bladder for relatively long periods of time. This, in turn, can be due to a number of factors:

- **Vesico-ureteric reflux** in which urine is refluxed back into the ureters. Around 40% of children with recurrent urinary tract infections are shown to have this defect on X-ray examination. The phenomenon is thought to have its origins in a congenital defect in the anatomy at the junction of the ureters into the bladder.
- Any **obstruction** to the normal outflow of urine from the bladder. **Folds**, or **valves**, in the urethra can be a factor causing this type of obstruction, as can **stones** in older children.

- **Incomplete emptying of the bladder,** due to haste, can also have a bearing on the amount of urine which remains in the bladder for long periods of time. Children are usually impatient of the need to empty their bladders and can be skilled at saying they have 'finished', when, in fact, a great quantity of urine can be remaining in the bladder. (Later, in schooldays, the bladder may be emptied infrequently – perhaps due to a dislike, or fear, of school toilets. This can cause the bladder to over-distend and subsequently to empty incompletely.)

The causative factors in the onset of urinary tract infections are complex and are intricately interwoven. Various tests, interpreted by skilled personnel, are necessary to unravel these factors in each individual child.

CHARACTERISTICS

Urinary tract infections are notoriously difficult to diagnose in children as signs and symptoms can be vague and non-specific, and often apparently unrelated to the urinary tract. The younger the child the more non-specific will be the symptoms.

Classically, the symptoms associated with a urinary tract infection are:

- **pain** on **passing urine** – a hot, burning sensation as the urine is voided;
- **pain** in either the **lower abdomen** – or higher up in the **loin** region if the infection has reached the kidneys – when it is known as a **pyelonephritis**;
- **frequency** in the passage of urine;
- **enuresis** and/or day-time wetting;
- the passage of **blood in the urine** (haematuria).

This picture is more usually seen in the older child with a urinary infection.

Younger children are more likely to be suffering from a urinary infection when:

- there is a **failure to gain weight** adequately;
- the child is generally **irritable**, and especially when this is also associated with a **poor appetite**;
- there is a **low-grade fever**, or spikes of fever perhaps with an associated febrile convulsion;
- **vomiting** can also occur with no previous obvious tummy upset.

Examination of a sample of urine will either confirm, or exclude, a urinary tract infection.

INVESTIGATIONS

In order to carry out a **urine test**, it is necessary that a clean sample (i.e. one that is not contaminated with either bacteria from the surrounding skin or by faeces) is obtained. To obtain a clean sample, the middle of the stream of urine should be taken. This is easier to obtain in boys than in girls without contamination. But with care, and after cleansing of the perineum, this can be obtained from a small girl as she sits on the pot or lavatory. Younger children can be fitted with a special bag until sufficient urine is obtained – again, of course, after thorough cleansing of the perineum.

The urine should be examined under the microscope as soon as possible after collection – within an hour if left unrefrigerated. (Refrigeration at 4°C for 24 hours is satisfactory for later laboratory examination.) Any pus cells, white blood cells and bacteria can be visualised under the microscope if they are present.

A further method – of value in the general practice situation – is to use a special **dip-slide**, which is a slide coated with a special culture medium. This slide is passed through the stream of urine and subsequently sent to the laboratory.

Blood tests will show a raised white blood cell count and ESR if an infection is present.

If urine testing proves infection to be the cause of the child's symptoms, further investigations (after the treatment of the acute attack) should be carried out in order to:

- see if the **kidneys** have been involved in this, or previous, infections;
- detect any **abnormalities in the renal tract**.

There are a number of specialised tests available. Different authorities usually have preference for one test over another. Also, the investigations pursued in the case of any one child will depend on the facilities available locally. These possible investigations include:

- **X-ray** examination of the abdomen. This, as a preliminary examination, will exclude any defects in the spine which may be a causative factor in the onset of the urinary tract infections. Any calcium stones in the urinary tract will also be shown up by this examination.
- **Ultra-sound** investigation. This can discern any obstructive problems as well as being of use in measuring bladder capacity and function.
- A **micturating cystogram** in which a radio-opaque dye is passed up into the bladder. As this is subsequently voided from the bladder, X-ray pictures are taken of the process. This is a particularly useful investigation in the detection of vesico-ureteric reflux. Also, any congenital kidney abnormalities – such as 'horse-shoe' or 'duplex' kidneys – will be detected. Again, the extent of any scarring of the kidneys, from previous infections, can be seen.

- **Isotope scanning** (DMSA scan) is a further investigation that is available at some centres. This specialised investigation is especially valuable in determining the presence and/or extent of kidney damage.
- **Intravenous urography** can also be used, and gives a comprehensive image of the structure and function of the whole urinary tract. This involves an intravenous injection of a radio-opaque substance.

Not all these investigations will, of course, be necessary in any one individual. Local availability, medical preference and the duration and severity of symptoms will all be taken into account when investigations are planned.

(Regretfully, child **sexual abuse** must always be remembered in children of all ages with recurrent urinary tract infections, and a watch must be kept for other signs and symptoms of this sad situation.)

MANAGEMENT

The acute attack

Babies and children with a severe urinary tract infection will need hospital treatment. Older children and those with a milder attack can be treated at home.

Antibiotics will need to be given as soon as possible. The choice of antibiotic will depend on the type of organism causing the infection. (It is not necessary, or wise, to await laboratory results before starting treatment. A wide spectrum antibiotic can be used until sensitivities are available. The type of antibiotic can always be changed if it is found that a different one is more appropriate for the specific infection.) Children who are seriously ill, or who are vomiting frequently, will need to be given antibiotics intravenously. Seven days of antibiotics should clear the infection.

Plenty of **fluids** – and an **analgesic** if pain is a problem – will help to lower temperature and reduce malaise. (Barley water, available in a variety of commercial flavours, is a useful and palatable drink to give to children. The urine is rendered less acid by these drinks, and provides a less advantageous medium for bacteria.)

'**Bubble bath**' **additives** should be avoided in the baths of children susceptible to urinary tract infections. The surface-tension lowering action of these additives aids the entry of bacteria into the bladder.

Future management will depend on the results of the investigations undertaken. For example, if any obstruction to the flow of urine, such as stones, is found, it will need to be dealt with.

Further infections must be prevented as far as possible to avoid long-term effects. This can be done by:

- giving a long-term dose of antibiotics. The length of time that these drugs should be given is variable, but a minimum of two years is advised by most authorities;
- being sure that the child empties his/her bladder fully. This can be helped by drinking plenty of water, allowing adequate time for visits to the lavatory and avoiding constipation – overloading of the large bowel can exert pressure on the lower urinary tract and effectively prevent adequate bladder emptying;
- assessing progress at follow-up appointments, with further investigative procedures when necessary. These procedures are vital to be sure that a low-grade infection does not persist, as well as to encourage child and parents to persist with treatment. (Long-term medication can be trying for everyone concerned.)

COMPLICATIONS

Recurrent urinary tract infections, with the continuing risk of further renal damage, is an ever present worry.

A long term effect, which will become evident in later life, is **renal failure** which occurs if damage has been severe in childhood. A **high blood pressure** can also be a late result of earlier kidney problems. **Kidney function** is intimately tied up with hypertension, but by early, adequate treatment of urinary tract infections in childhood at least one possible cause of this problem can be eliminated.

Urinary tract infections in childhood are an excellent example of how adult disease often has its basis in the early growing years.

WARTS

Verrucas.

INCIDENCE

Warts are common skin lesions and especially so during childhood. In fact, almost all children will have warts somewhere on their bodies before adulthood is reached.

Verrucas, or plantar warts, which are found on children's feet, reach almost epidemic proportions at times. This type of wart is rarely seen after the age of 16 years.

HISTORY

Warts have been referred to in history from time immemorial. Probably one of the best known characters in British history with facial warts is Oliver Cromwell, who had a splendid crop. It is only in recent years that a greater interest has been shown in these benign tumours of the skin. The causative factor – a particular type of virus – is known and is seen to multiply rapidly in the nuclei of cells. It is recognized that, under certain circumstances, infection with one of the viruses causing warts can lead to malignant change. Further study of warts may help to unravel aspects of malignancies in the body.

CAUSATION

Warts are caused by one of the Papilloma viruses – of which there are many – of the Papova group. It is thought that the incubation period (the period between infection and the appearance of the wart) is long.

CHARACTERISTICS

Four different types of wart are described and, although these can overlap, it is possible that a different type of subgroup of virus is involved in each type.

The **common wart** or **verruca vulgaris** is most usually seen over bony surfaces such as knees and elbows. It is possible that small, regular episodes of minor injury to these parts of the body allow the virus to gain a hold. These warts are raised and under a magnifying lens can be seen to have an irregular, bumpy surface.

Plane warts are, as their name implies, flat and are usually found on exposed parts of the body, particularly the face. They are also seen to occur along the margins of scratches and cuts – frequently in large numbers.

Plantar warts – usually referred to merely as 'verrucas' – are found on the soles of the feet. Over recent years much publicity has been given to this type of wart because of the high number of children acquiring verrucas from swimming pools, and also following barefoot exercise and dancing. They can become large and exceedingly painful from the trauma of continually walking on them.

Warts around the anus and genital regions of the body tend to have a frilly, fronded appearance. Sexual abuse must always be borne in mind when a child is found to have warts on this part of the body.

MANAGEMENT

This can be fraught with difficulties due to a number of factors:

- the position of the warts – for example, numerous plane warts on the face can be very difficult to treat; plantar warts, too, can be numerous and cover a large, much-used part of the foot; numerous warts on fingers can also cause problems by getting in the way of fine, delicate activities;
- the fact that warts frequently occur in groups, making treatment difficult;
- warts quickly appear out of the blue, and at times disappear with equal rapidity. (Many are the old wives' tales connected with this phenomenon – one of the best-known being that if you rub the wart with raw steak and then bury the steak in the garden, as the meat degenerates, so, too, will the wart disappear!)

Specific treatments include the following.

- **Paints**, which basically remove hard skin, can be applied to the wart on a regular daily basis. It is preferable that the painted area is covered by a plaster dressing to avoid the paint being rubbed off. This treatment will need to be continued for some time, and frequently fails because of this need for long-term treatment.
- **Podophyllin** can be used for single – or if there are only a few – warts. Again, this should be applied daily and covered with a dressing. This substance must be used with caution, however, as it is extremely irritant when applied to normal skin. Between applications, the surface of the wart can be gently rubbed away.

Both the above preparations can be bought over the counter in main chemists.

- **Carbon dioxide 'snow'** or **liquid nitrogen** can also be used for isolated warts. Again, it is important that the wart should be treated accurately, as surrounding normal skin can be easily damaged.
- Soaking the feet daily in a solution of **formaldehyde** used to be a favourite treatment. Following each 'soak', the surface of the wart was gently pared away. Once again this is slow, long-term treatment and is rarely used today.
- Warts can be **cauterized**. A little local anaesthetic is injected around the wart and the warty tissue is burnt away. Care must be taken not to damage the surrounding skin. It is unwise to use this method for warts arising over joints or on the palms of the hands or soles of the feet. The resultant scars can be painful in these specific locations.
- A simple, but often effective, method for the solitary wart is merely to cover it with an **airtight plaster**. This effectively cuts off the oxygen supply to the wart. After 2 or 3 weeks of this treatment – changing the plaster at bath-times, or as and when it becomes dirty or loose – the wart will become soft and friable. It can then be gently scrubbed off with pumice or an ordinary nail-brush.

PREVENTION

Preventative methods are only possible with plantar warts – the ubiquitous verrucas that are passed so readily from child to child in the warm, moist atmosphere of swimming pools. A few authorities still inspect children's feet before swimming and follow this by exclusion from the baths of those children found to have a verruca. This is difficult to implement fully, and perhaps not entirely reasonable to enforce. No child ever died from a verruca, but many children have lost their lives through being unable to swim. **Verruca socks** have had their vogue in the past and are still available. Children don these foot coverings before entering the changing room (where most of the infections are passed on) of swimming pools.

Warts have a nuisance value rather than being dangerous. But there are occasions when treatment for these irritating lesions becomes necessary. Painful verrucas on feet, disfiguring marks on the face or warts on fingers getting in the way of daily activities are all examples of reasons for active treatment. But even with conscientious treatment, warts can be particularly persistent. Their only saving grace is that they will eventually disappear spontaneously within a year or two if left alone!

Whooping-cough

Alternative names

Pertussis; the 'cough of a hundred days'.

Incidence

The incidence of whooping-cough in England and Wales has shown a marked variation over the past 25 years. This is closely related to the up-take of whooping-cough vaccine, the incidence being dramatically increased when immunization rates were low, and falling again as immunization against this vicious disease became more acceptable.

Pertussis (whooping-cough) is known worldwide, and estimated figures in 1986 were 60 million cases in a year. Half a million deaths annually were also reported at this time. Without immunization, it is thought that by the age of 5 years 80% of children are infected.

Whooping-cough is unusual among the childhood infections in being more common in girls, and also of greater severity.

Epidemics of this infection occur once every 3–4 years. This has been noted both in the UK and in other countries where reports of infectious disease are relatively reliable. (It is thought that whooping-cough is under-reported in most countries where standardized reporting systems are in place. So the true incidence of this disease is probably very high indeed.) This 3–4-year pattern was noticed again in the UK when the immunization figures fell to a low level in the 1970s. During the 10 years or so that it took for the immunization levels to rise again, two epidemics were noted – in 1978–1979 and in 1982–1983. In both these periods over 400 000 cases were notified.

Causation

Whooping-cough is caused by a bacterium. This bacterium is spread by droplet infection from a child already suffering from the disease.

The mode of action of the whooping-cough bacterium (*Bordetella pertussis*) is unusual. The bacterium itself first of all attacks the respiratory passages, producing the initial symptoms of the disease, which are rather similar to those of a common cold. The bacterium then produces a toxin which attacks various cells throughout the body. So while the initial bacterial attack is susceptible to, and can be treated with, antibiotics, these drugs will have no effect on the later toxin.

The incubation period of whooping-cough is 7–14 days – 10 days being the average time before the next family member starts to show symptoms.

CHARACTERISTICS

Whooping-cough is a long illness, with three distinct phases.

- During the **catarrhal stage**, symptoms closely akin to a common cold occur – a **runny nose**, a **cough** and a **mild fever**. This stage can be so comparatively mild that the child may still be at school or playing with his/her peers. As s/he is infectious at this time, the disease can be quickly spread.
- The **paroxysmal stage** follows after about 10 days. This is when the cough occurs in severe spasms and the child has great difficulty in getting adequate breath between the paroxysms. The face will become puce and even blue with the effort to get air into the lungs, and the paroxysm will end in a 'whoop' as the air is finally drawn in a rush into the lungs. Once heard, the 'whoop' of whooping-cough can never again be forgotten. **Vomiting** frequently occurs at the end of the paroxysm of coughing, particularly if the child has just eaten.

  These paroxysmal attacks are extremely distressing to both parent and child. With closely repeated paroxysms the whole family – and especially the sufferer – can become completely exhausted. This phase can last up to a fortnight.

  The lack of oxygen experienced by the child during these paroxysms of coughing can be the cause of one of the most serious of the complications seen due to whooping-cough. The severity of the paroxysms can result in **haemorrhages** into various parts of the body – into the conjunctiva of the eyes, from the nose and even small bleeding areas into the skin.
- During the **convalescent stage** the cough gradually decreases in both frequency and severity, but can still be in evidence up to 3 months later – hence 'the hundred-day cough'.

If the disease occurs in a young baby, the characteristic 'whoop' is often absent. At this age the baby will not have the strength to take the large gasp that is the cause of the typical 'whoop'.

INVESTIGATIONS

The diagnosis of whooping-cough is essentially a clinical one, and a very obvious one once the 'whoop' is heard. If there is a current epidemic of whooping-cough and a child has a persistent, worsening cough lasting for longer than 2 weeks, whooping-cough can be strongly suspected.

Blood tests will show a non-specific increase in certain of the white blood cells.

Laboratory tests on the secretions obtained from the back of the nose and throat can confirm the diagnosis. This, however, is rarely done, partly because of the unpleasantness for the child of the procedure involved in obtaining a sample of these secretions, and partly because of the unreliability of some of these tests.

MANAGEMENT

A specific antibiotic, **erythromycin**, is given to destroy the bacteria (but with no action against the toxin produced). This treatment will also render the child non-infectious after around 5 days. The erythromycin should be continued for 2 weeks to be sure of eradicating all the bacteria.

During the unpleasant paroxysmal phase, the child can be helped in a number of ways.

- Efforts should be made to **avoid provoking the paroxysms** of cough-ing. For example, sudden changes of temperature can initiate an at-tack, so nursing in a warm, evenly controlled environment can be helpful. Similarly, bland food that does not irritate the back of the child's throat should be offered.
- **Meals should be small and frequent**. If a fit of coughing results in vomiting, with the loss of most of the previous meal, food can be of-fered again once the attack is over. (Unlike after the vomiting due to a tummy upset, the child will often be willing to eat again immedi-ately after an attack of coughing.) It is important to do everything possible to maintain the child's nutrition during the illness. Fluids should also be available in abundance to be sure that dehydration does not complicate the illness.
- The **sticky mucus**, production of which is part of this disease, **must be removed** from the child's respiratory passages as much as possible. This is especially important in babies and young children, who find it difficult, or impossible, to cough up this mucus. (This aspect is one of the reasons why whooping-cough is such a dangerous illness in the young child.)
- Children with whooping-cough can become very distressed and frightened during the paroxysms of coughing (as can the adults watching their child fighting for breath) and will need much **reassurance**.

Most older children can be **nursed at home** through an attack of whooping-cough. Young babies, or those children in difficult or unsuit-able home circumstances, will need to be **admitted to hospital** during the worst of the illness. Hospital admission for a short time may also be neces-sary to relieve parents who are nursing several children through this long-drawn-out illness.

School can be recommended as soon as the child feels well enough – as long as at least 5 days treatment with erythromycin has been given. It is un-likely, however, that the child will feel well enough to return to school for **at least 2 or 3 weeks** with even a mild attack of whooping-cough. Teachers should be fully informed about the **course of the illness** – mainly because the cough, which can last for up to 3 months, can give rise to concern. Teaching staff should be reassured that **the child is not infectious** during this convalescent stage as long as erythromycin has been given.

COMPLICATIONS

As well as being a highly unpleasant, and potentially fatal, illness, complications are common with an attack of whooping-cough.

Lungs

Bronchopneumonia not infrequently occurs along with an attack of whooping-cough. Resistance is lowered by the effects of the whooping-cough bacteria and the toxin produced, so that secondary infection is common. If this occurs the child's general condition will deteriorate and there will be a rise in temperature. Treatment will be with a further antibiotic.

Children who suffer from **asthma** will have added problems if they contract whooping-cough. Indeed this infection may bring a hitherto undiagnosed asthma to light. Once recovery from the whooping-cough has occurred, appropriate treatment for the asthma must be given (see Asthma, above). Some authorities consider that an attack of whooping cough in childhood contributes to long-term damage to the lungs – **bronchiectasis** being a common sequel. Appropriate antibiotic treatment during the acute attack will do much to reduce this possibility.

Ears

Secondary bacterial infection giving rise to **otitis media** is frequently found to occur during the acute stages of whooping-cough. Earache and a rise in temperature will alert to this complication.

Haemorrhages

Because of the excessive strain put on blood vessels during the paroxysms of coughing, haemorrhages into various parts of the body can readily occur. **Conjunctival haemorrhages, petechiae** (bleeding from small blood vessels under the skin) and **nose-bleeds** have already been mentioned. **Coughing up of blood** from the respiratory passages can also occur and add to parental anxieties. These haemorrhages will all resolve spontaneously, although nose-bleeding can sometimes be a problem to control. Haemoptysis (coughing up of blood) should always be reported to the doctor.

Hernias

Again because of the severity of the paroxysmal attacks of coughing, the pressure inside the abdominal cavity is raised. If there is already a hernia present – in boys most usually in the groin area – or there is an incipient weakness in the muscles in this part of the body, an attack of whooping-cough can bring this to light.

Nervous system

It is the complications in the nervous system due to the whooping-cough bacteria that are the most serious. These complications can result in long-term handicap. It is thought that there are two ways in which these complications can occur:

- as a result of the temporary oxygen lack to the tissues, including nervous tissue, from the paroxysms of coughing – anyone who has seen the cyanosis (blueness) of a child's face during a paroxysm will readily understand how tissues are starved of oxygen during those few minutes;
- as a direct result of the effects of the toxin produced by the whooping-cough bacteria on nervous tissue.

These neurological complications can manifest themselves as **convulsions** or **loss of consciousness**. If severe, the outcome can be **permanent brain damage**, resulting in a range of possible effects, including **paralysis, intellectual handicap** and **death**.

Regretfully, there is no treatment that can prevent such tragedies occurring, apart from, of course, earlier prevention by immunization with whooping-cough vaccine.

PREVENTION

Whooping-cough can be prevented by **immunization** with whooping-cough vaccine. This vaccine is offered, in the UK, as part of the routine babyhood immunization schedule. This schedule is for whooping-cough vaccine to be given together with vaccines against diphtheria and tetanus as the '**triple' vaccine** at 2, 3 and 4 months of age. If the whooping-cough part of this triple vaccine has been missed out for any reason, it can be given as three doses of single whooping-cough vaccine at monthly intervals.

Contraindications to receiving this vaccine are few.

- If the child has a feverish illness when any immunization procedures are due, they should be postponed until recovery has taken place, and this, of course, applies to the whooping-cough vaccine as much as to any other.
- If there has been a **severe** generalized reaction to a previous dose of the whooping-cough vaccine, this part of the triple vaccine should be omitted in future. A severe reaction means a high fever (over 39.5°C) within 48 hours of the injection; convulsions, anaphylactic shock or prolonged, inconsolable screaming by the baby within 72 hours of the injection being given – all pretty dramatic occurrences, which should not be confused with mild reactions, such as a mild fever or irritability for a few hours. These latter mild reactions can occur following immunization with the whooping-cough vaccine. But when compared with the possible effects of a naturally acquired attack of whooping-cough, the benefits of immunization can be seen.
- A **severe** local reaction to a previous immunization at the site of the actual injection is a contraindication. This means a large area of

redness and swelling – covering the front and side of the baby's thigh or much of the circumference of the arm, depending on where the injection has been given.

Asthma or eczema are not contraindications to receiving the whooping-cough vaccine, and no child should be denied the protection of this vaccine because s/he suffers from these conditions.

If the baby has had any convulsions earlier in life, or there is a strong history of epilepsy in the immediate family, individual advice regarding this must be taken from a doctor specializing in immunization problems.

THE FUTURE

For the individual, the late effects of an attack of whooping-cough will depend on any complications that may have occurred. For most children an attack of whooping-cough will be a dim, distant, albeit unpleasant, memory. But for some unfortunate children, this infection will colour the whole of the rest of their lives.

APPENDIX A: THE PROGRESS OF INFECTIOUS DISEASES (UNCOMPLICATED)

INTRODUCTION

It must be emphasized that, as no two people are the same and the same disease affects people in different ways, the following information should only be treated as a guide.

CHICKENPOX

Days	Stage	Comments
	Incubation	14–17 days' duration
1–5	Rash crops	Crops of 'blistery' spots arise every 2–3 days
1–6	Fever	Usually peaks on third day – can be up to 39°C
6–9	Rash scabs	Spots crust over

NB. All stages of the rash can be seen at the same time.

MEASLES

Days	Stage	Comments
	Incubation	10–14 days' duration
1–7	Conjunctivitis	Sore reddened eyes associated with photophobia
1–7	Fever	Up to 40°C – usually peaks on fourth day
1–7	Coryza	Runny nose
1–11	Cough	Harsh dry cough
2–6	Koplik's spots	To be found on inside of cheeks opposite the back molars – similar to grains of salt
4–9	Rash – discrete	Face, upper torso and arms – becoming a confluent dense rash all over the body after about 1–3 days

RUBELLA

Days	Stage	Comments
	Incubation	14–21 days' duration
1–8	Malaise	
1–12	Lymph nodes	Tender enlarged glands at back of neck
4–7	Conjunctivitis	Mild only, with no photophobia
4–7	Coryza	Runny nose
4–7	Rash	Fine, pink discrete spots
5–8	Fever	Mild only, but may be up to 38°C on fifth day

SCARLET FEVER

Days	Stage	Comments
	Incubation	2–4 days' duration
1–5	Sore throat	Severe sore throat
2–7	Fever	Can be up to 40°C on third day
2–7	Rash	Bright scarlet in colour

Appendix B: GLOSSARY

Abdominal cavity That part of the torso below the diaphragm, containing many important organs

Aetiology The cause of, or factors involved in, the onset of a disease

Alveoli Lung tissue involved in gaseous exchange

Anal fissure Crack in skin around anus

Analgesics Pain-relieving drugs

Androgens Male sex hormones

Aneurysm Ballooning of an artery

Anorexia Loss of appetite

Antibiotics Drugs active against bacterial infections

Anus Ring of muscular tissue at lower end of large bowel

Auroscope Instrument used for examining ears

Bronchiolitis An infection in the smallest bronchi in the lungs

Capillaries The smallest blood vessels in the body

Cataract Clouding of the lens of the eye

Cellulitis Widespread inflammation of connective tissue

Cerebrospinal fluid Fluid surrounding the brain and spinal cord

Chorea Involuntary, non-stereotyped muscular movements

Chromosomes Units in every cell on which genes are situated

Chronic Long-standing

Comedones Plugs of hard skin found in acne

Congenital Conditions existing from birth

Conjunctiva Delicate tissue covering the eye

Conjunctivitis Inflammation of the conjunctiva

Connective tissue Tissues surrounding all the organs of the body

Constitutional upset Generalized illness, usually with fever and malaise

CT scan Computer-aided tomography

Desquamation Peeling of the superficial layers of the skin

Developmental checks Standardized tests used to check childhood development

Diaphragm Strong sheet of muscle dividing the abdominal cavity from the chest cavity

Dietician Person trained in nutrition

Droplet infection Spread of infection from minute drops of secretions in a person's breath

EEG Electroencephalogram

Elimination diets Diets used to exclude possible cause of an allergy

Emollient creams Greasy ointments or creams used in skin diseases

Encephalitis Inflammation of the brain

Epicanthic folds Folds of skin over inner corner of some children's eyes

Epiglottis   Flap of tissue at the back of the throat controlling respiration and swallowing

Epiglottitis   Infection of the epiglottis

Epistaxis   Nose bleeding

Erythromycin   A particular type of antibiotic

ESR   (Erythrocyte sedimentation rate) – laboratory test used as an indicator of an infective process

Eustachian tube   Tiny tube linking the middle ear with the back of the throat

Febrile convulsions   Convulsions (fits or seizures) seen in children under the age of 5 years due to a sudden rise in temperature

Glaucoma   Condition in which pressure inside the eye is raised

Glycosuria   Sugar in the urine

Haemangioma   A naevus due to an underlying abnormality in the blood vessels

Haematuria   Blood in the urine

Haemoglobin   Substance in red blood cells carrying oxygen

Haemophilia   Condition associated with defective clotting of blood

Haemoptysis   Coughing up of blood

Hernia   Weakness in muscular wall – usually of abdomen

Hirschsprung's disease   Condition in which there are narrowed segments of bowel

Hormones   Secretions from ductless glands that are poured directly into the blood stream

Hypertrophy   Enlargement of a part of the body

Hypoglycaemia   Low blood sugar

Hypothermia   Low body temperature

Immunization   Procedures eliciting a response in the body that protects against specific infections met at a later date

Immunosuppression   A procedure whereby the immune system is suppressed by drugs in the treatment of certain diseases

Incubation period   That period of time between exposure to an infection and the onset of symptoms

Inhaler   Specialized equipment used to introduce medication into the lungs

Jaundice   Yellow coloration of the skin due to malfunction of the liver

Ketones   Substances that can arise from the breakdown of body tissue

Koplik spots   Spots seen on inside of cheeks in the early stages of measles

Labyrinthitis   Inflammation of structures inside the ears due to infection, causing giddiness

Lumbar puncture   Procedure whereby cerebrospinal fluid is withdrawn for diagnostic purposes

Lymph nodes   Congregation of lymph tissue in many different parts of the body

Malaise   General feeling of illness

Mastoid process   Bony projection of skull behind and below the ears

Menarche   Time of onset of menstruation in girls at puberty

Meninges   Thin, delicate covering of brain and spinal cord

Meningitis   Inflammation of meninges

Myringotomy   Procedure whereby an opening is made in the eardrum to withdraw fluid from the middle ear

Naevi   Specific types of skin blemish

Nebulizer   Equipment for introducing medication into the lungs by way of a face mask

Oestrogens   Female sex hormones

Orchitis   Inflammation of the testes

Ossicles   Tiny bones in the middle ear – three in number

Osteoporosis   Reduction in density of bones

Pancreatitis   Inflammation of the pancreas

Parasite   An organism living off another unrelated organism

Parotid glands   Salivary glands situated in front of, and below, the ears

Parotitis   Inflammation of the parotid salivary glands

Petechiae   Small bleeding points under the skin

Photophobia   Dislike of light

Pica   Eating of dirt, or other unsuitable substances, e.g. coal, chalk

Platelets   Part of the blood concerned with clotting

Psychiatrist   A doctor specializing in mental illness

Refractive error   Errors in the bending of light on to the retina

Renal tract   Organs of excretion, consisting of kidneys, ureters, bladder and urethra

Retina   The structure at the back of the eye intimately concerned with vision

Rheumatoid factor   Factor found in the blood of sufferers from some kinds of rheumatism or arthritis

Rickets   Disease of bone due to lack of calcium and/or vitamin D

Scoliosis   Sideways twist to the spine

Sebaceous glands   Glands found all over the body producing sebum, which gives the skin its oily nature

Septicaemia   Blood poisoning

Signing   Language using hand movements for deaf people

Soft palate   Back of the roof of the mouth

Syndrome   A combination of signs and symptoms which, when put together, form a recognizable pattern

Thrush   A fungal yeast infection

Tonsils   Aggregations of lymphoid tissue on either side of the throat

Toxin   Substance produced by certain bacteria

Trachea   Windpipe

Ureters   Tubes connecting kidneys to bladder

Urethra   Passage from bladder to exterior

Vasculitis   Inflammation of the small blood vessels

APPENDIX C: IMMUNIZATION

Immunization against some of the common childhood infectious fevers is one of the success stories of the 20th century. Before this children had to suffer a naturally acquired attack (usually caught from another child) so that their immune systems could develop antibodies against the infection. With immunization procedures, the need to contract the specific infections (with all the attendant risks of complications and even death) is by-passed. Laboratory methods are available to modify the viruses and bacteria causing disease. This means that an immune response is possible without the toxic components of the infection that give rise to the unpleasant, and potentially fatal, symptoms of the naturally acquired infection.

There are two main forms of immunization – active immunization and passive immunization. By far the most commonly used method is active immunization, where modified organisms are injected (or given by mouth in the case of the polio immunization). This stimulates the baby's immune system to produce antibodies against the specific organism that has been injected. These antibodies are then available to fight any future invasions of the body by the specific organisms.

Passive immunization is used less frequently and consists of an injection already containing antibodies. This type of immunization is used for short-term protection, such as overseas travel, or for children whose immune system is compromised by an existing condition or by drugs to treat some other serious disease.

In the UK there are routine procedures for the immunization of all babies:

- at 2, 3 and 4 months – diphtheria/tetanus/whooping-cough (pertussis) by injection as a combined vaccine; also at this time the oral polio vaccine is given as well as the injection against *Haemophilus influenzae* type b;
- at 12–15 months – measles/mumps/rubella by injection as a combined vaccine;
- at 3–5 years – booster doses of diphtheria/tetanus and oral polio; a booster measles/mumps/rubella injection is also given;
- at 13–15 years – booster doses of tetanus and oral polio are given.

BCG vaccine is also given between the ages of 10–14 years as protection against tuberculosis. Before this vaccine is given a skin test (the Heaf test) is done to determine whether or not the child has already acquired some immunity against tuberculosis. Very few children these days have this acquired immunity, so most will need the BCG vaccine.

On occasions this vaccine is given in early infancy if the baby is thought to be at special risk of contracting tuberculosis.

The diseases against which immunization is available are potentially fatal and can leave behind serious long-term handicap. So while there are a few risks in immunization procedures, the benefits are enormous. Risks are reduced to an absolute minimum if the following contraindications to receiving the vaccine are observed:

- if the baby has an acute illness (immunization needs to be postponed until the infection has cleared);
- if there has been a severe reaction to a previous immunization;
- if the baby has a condition in which the immune system is deficient; similarly, if the baby/child needs special medication to suppress the immune system for some other cause;
- if the baby has been born with a severe condition affecting the central nervous system.

Parents need to discuss with the person giving the immunization if they have any worries at all about whether their child should receive the immunization.

Reactions to vaccines are unusual and vary very much in severity. These range from redness and swelling at the site of the injection or a mild fever to excessive crying or a convulsion. Medical advice must be taken for serious reactions, and further immunizations discussed fully.

Immunization is an enormous and complex subject, and only a brief outline can be given here. For further detailed information, textbooks on immunization should be studied or the Department of Health publication *Immunisation against Infectious Disease*.

As the infections against which immunization is available are seen only infrequently these days, a brief word about their signs and symptoms might be useful.

Tetanus is a severe disease affecting muscles, which contract into painful spasms, and when this affects the muscles of breathing it can be fatal. Once the toxin released by the organism has entered the body there is no available treatment. Tetanus is acquired from spores found in the earth, which can enter the body via the smallest cut or graze. It cannot be passed from person to person.

Poliomyelitis is caused by a virus that attacks nervous tissue and can cause permanent paralysis. (The descriptive name for polio that was in common use in the early 20th century was 'infantile paralysis', and created much fear – understandably – in parents' minds.) If the muscles of respiration are affected the infection can be fatal – or else the sufferer will need respiratory help throughout his/her life. Milder attacks did occur without paralysis, but the risk was always a worrying possibility.

As late as 1955 there were 4000 cases of paralytic polio in the UK. Following mass immunization there were only 28 cases reported between 1985 and 1994.

Haemophilus influenzae type b (Hib) is an important cause of meningitis in the under-4s. Following the routine immunization of babies there has been a marked decline in meningitis due to this cause. (It must be remembered, however, that there are a number of other organisms that can cause meningitis.)

Details of diphtheria, whooping-cough, measles, mumps and rubella can be found in other parts of this volume.

Further reading

Carson, P. (1987) *Coping Successfully with Your Child's Asthma*, Sheldon Press, London.

David, T. J. (ed.) (1992) *Recent Advances in Paediatrics*, Churchill Livingstone, Edinburgh.

Department of Health, Welsh Office (1996) *Immunisation against Infectious Disease*, HMSO, London.

Elliot, J. (1987) *If Your Child is Diabetic*, Sheldon Press, London.

Forfar, J. O. (ed.) (1988) *Child Health in a Changing Society*, Oxford University Press, Oxford.

Green, C. (1997) *Toddler Taming – a Parent's Guide to the First 4 Years*, Vermilion, London.

Hall, D. M. B. (1989) *Health for All Children*, Oxford Medical Publishers, Oxford.

Hollyer, B. and Smith, L. (1996) *Sleep – the Secret of Peaceful Nights*, Ward Lock, London.

Hospital for Sick Children (1997) *The Great Ormond Street New Book of Baby and Child Care*, Vermilion, London.

Knight, A. (1981) *Asthma and Hay-fever*, Positive Health Guides, London.

Lewis, S. and National Eczema Society (1994) *The Eczema Handbook*, Vermilion, London.

Nicoll, A. (ed.) (1989) *Manual on Infections and Immunisations in Children*, Oxford Medical Publications, Oxford.

Palmar, R. L. (1989) *Anorexia Nervosa*, Penguin Books, London.

Polney, L. (1989) *Manual of Community Paediatrics*, Churchill Livingstone, Edinburgh.

Reisner, H. (1987) *Children with Epilepsy*, Woodbine House, Rockville, USA.

Rossiter, J. and Seddon, R. (1992) *Diabetic Kid's Cookbook*, Positive Health Guides, London.

Taitz, L. S. and Wardley, B. (1989) *Handbook of Child Nutrition*, Oxford Medical Publishers, Oxford.

van Riel, P. (1987) *Acne*, Sheldon Press, London.

INDEX